It Happened to Me

Series Editor: Arlene Hirschfelder

Books in the "It Happened to Me" series are designed for inquisitive teens digging for answers about certain illnesses, social issues, or lifestyle interests. Whether you are deep into your teen years or just entering them, these books are gold mines of up-to-date information, riveting teen views, and great visuals to help you figure out stuff. Besides special boxes highlighting singular facts, each book is enhanced with the latest reading list, web sites, and an index. Perfect for browsing, there's loads of expert information by acclaimed writers to help parents, guardians, and librarians understand teen illness, tough situations, and lifestyle choices.

Epilepsy

The Ultimate Teen Guide

KATHLYN GAY
AND SEAN MCGARRAHAN

It Happened to Me, No. 2

The Scarecrow Press, Inc.
Lanham, Maryland • Toronto • Plymouth, UK

SCARECROW PRESS, INC.

Published in the United States of America
by Scarecrow Press, Inc.
A wholly owned subsidiary of
The Rowman & Littlefield Publishing Group, Inc.
4501 Forbes Boulevard, Suite 200, Lanham, Maryland 20706
www.scarecrowpress.com

Estover Road
Plymouth PL6 7PY
United Kingdom

British Library Cataloguing in Publication Information Available

The hardback edition of this book was previously cataloged by the Library of Congress
as follows:

Gay, Kathlyn.
    Epilepsy : the ultimate teen guide / Kathlyn Gay and Sean McGarrahan.
        v. cm. — (It happened to me)
    Includes index.
    Contents: 1. What's epilepsy? 2. Fact or folklore? 3. What's happening? 4. Diagnosis and
treatment 5. Surgery for epilepsy 6. Living with epilepsy 7. School and job issues 8. Sports and
recreation 9. The female factor 10. Finding a cure.
    ISBN 0-8108-4339-0
    1. Epilepsy in adolescence—Juvenile literature. 2. Epilepsy—Juvenile literature. [1. Epilepsy.
2. Diseases.] I. McGarrahan, Sean II. Title. III. Series

    RJ496.E6 G39 2002
    616.8'53'0835—dc21   2002004718

ISBN: 0-8108-4339-0 (hardcover)
ISBN: 978-0-8108-5835-0 / 0-8108-5835-5 (paperback)

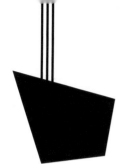

Contents

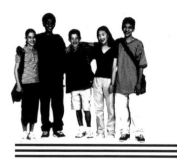

Contents

Acknowledgments

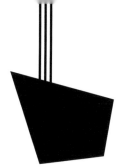

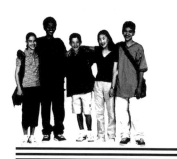

A special thank you to Jerome Engel Jr., M.D., Ph.D., Professor Departments of Neurology and Neurobiology, Director UCLA Seizure Disorders Center, for reviewing our book manuscript for accuracy and offering helpful suggestions; we greatly appreciate his concerns and efforts. Another special thanks is due Susan S. Spencer, M.D., Professor of Neurology, Yale University School of Medicine, for her time and efforts preparing MRI print images for use in this book.

We are also grateful for the stories and experiences that teenagers and others have shared regarding their seizures. And we especially commend those who work to make the general public aware of epilepsy and its impact on people with the disorder and their families, friends, and associates.

Thank you, also, to Arlene Hirschfelder, series editor, for her many helpful suggestions and guidance in preparing the manuscript for this book.

Kathlyn Gay and Sean McGarrahan

1 What's Epilepsy?

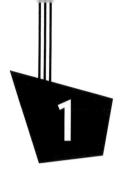

When you hear or read the term *epilepsy*, you aren't likely to associate it with these names:

- ○ Contemporary American actor Danny Glover
- ○ 1990s Scottish Paralympic multiple medal winner Margaret McEleney
- ○ Contemporary Canadian rock musician Neil Young
- ○ World famous screen and stage star Richard Burton
- ○ Early-twentieth-century comedian Bud Abbott of the Abbott and Costello team
- ○ Nineteenth-century Italian violinist Niccolo Paganini
- ○ Nineteenth-century American author Edgar Allan Poe
- ○ Nineteenth-century British author Charles Dickens
- ○ Seventeenth-century French scientist and mathematician Blaise Pascal
- ○ Fifteenth-century military leader and heroine Joan of Arc
- ○ Ancient Roman ruler Julius Caesar
- ○ Ancient Greek mathematician Pythagoras

Epilepsy is a brain disorder in which clusters of nerve cells, or neurons, in the brain sometimes signal abnormally.

—National Institute of Neurological Disorders and Stroke, National Institutes of Health

These famous people represent many walks of life, varied accomplishments, and different time periods, but they have something in common. They are among the millions today and yesterday who live or once lived with a brain disorder known as epilepsy.

At least 50 million people worldwide have epilepsy, and the disorder affects about 2.5 million Americans. Each year between 150,000 and 200,000 new cases occur in the United States. Most people with epilepsy are not famous, although they may have achieved a great deal in their lives.

A person with epilepsy could be a successful teacher, a computer specialist, a research physicist, a baseball player, a competitive swimmer, a musician, or an accomplished person in almost any other field. That goes for teenagers, too. A young person with epilepsy could be one of the most outstanding students in her or his school.

Did you know? Four to five of every 1,000 young people age eighteen and under in the United States have epilepsy. The number is about the same for those age eighteen to forty-five.

Yet people with epilepsy seldom want others to know about their condition, especially after the initial diagnosis. Why? Because epilepsy carries a stigma, which is a result of numerous myths, misconceptions, and misunderstandings that have prevailed for several thousand years and are unfortunately still widespread. In her book *Seizure Free,* Leanne Chilton explained that after she was first diagnosed with epilepsy, she hated telling anyone about it. "To have to tell an instructor or a student or a co-worker or anyone that I had epilepsy was a nightmare. . . . I felt like I was disclosing the most secret part of my entire life and then hoping to God that no one would take advantage of my vulnerability. . . . I always had this fear that once [people] found out, my life would end."[1]

Young people diagnosed with epilepsy often fear they are going to die or that they will suffer brain damage. Some may become depressed, extremely angry, or defiant.

To counter all the misinformation about this brain disorder, health care practitioners and groups worldwide try to educate the public as well as patients about epilepsy. First, it's important to note that epilepsy is not a single set of symptoms with specific characteristics. Rather, many different types of epilepsy have been diagnosed. In general, though, there are both primary and secondary partial epilepsies, and primary and secondary generalized epilepsies.

WHAT IS EPILEPSY?

"There are many types of epilepsy. Each type of epilepsy has different behavioral effects and is treated with different methods."

—Neuroscience for Kids

"Epilepsy is a physical illness which causes recurrent, sudden, brief changes in the normal electrical activity of the brain. During an episode of epilepsy, often called a 'seizure,' brain cells fire uncontrollably at up to four times their normal rate, temporarily affecting the way a person behaves, moves, thinks, or feels."

—inteliHealth

"Epilepsy is a tendency to have recurrent seizures. Seizures are episodes of disorganized electrical activity in the brain that can produce a broad spectrum of signs and symptoms, ranging from involuntary movements to loss of consciousness."

—Richard Lechtenberg, M.D.

Epilepsy is "a set of symptoms associated with abnormal nerve cell activity in the brain. . . . Instead of small bursts of electrical impulses, a group of nerve cells fires a storm of strong bursts like a platoon of soldiers all firing at once. Moreover, the firing comes with machine-gun rapidity."

—Johns Hopkins Medical Handbook

"Every individual with epileptic seizures is unique and . . . no single strategy—or even a medication—works for everyone."

—Robert Efron, M.D.,
School of Medicine, University of California, Davis

3

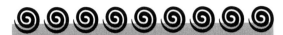

DENDRITES AND AXONS

Neurons consist of a cell body (1) that contains the nucleus, where most of the molecules that the neuron needs to survive and function are manufactured. Dendrites (2) extend out from the cell body like the branches of a tree and receive messages from other nerve cells. Signals then pass from the dendrites through the cell body and may travel away from the cell body down an axon (3) to another neuron, a muscle cell, or cells in some other organ. The neuron is usually surrounded by many support cells. Some types of cells wrap around the axon to form an insulating sheath (4).

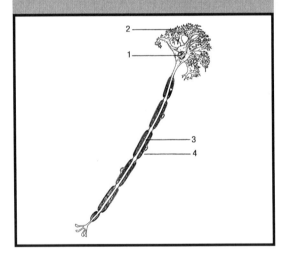

BRAIN CELLS

The human brain contains about 100 billion microscopic units called neurons, or nerve cells. Each nerve cell can produce and transmit electrical signals, and all are linked together in a complex network that allows the brain to do its work.

Although nerve cells do not touch each other, one neuron can communicate with or stimulate another through an electrical-chemical process. Electrical impulses begin "firing" or discharging to send messages. An impulse travels from one cell to another through *axons* and *dendrites* (from the Greek word *dendron,* meaning tree).

Axons are cablelike structures that carry information away from a cell and dendrites are like tiny tentacles that receive and deliver signals. Chemicals called neurotransmitters direct electrical impulses across a gap, known as a *synapse,* between nerve cells. The receiving cell has receptors that are activated and can "excite" or inhibit the neuron. If the nerve cell is excited (or stimulated), it fires a signal and the process continues. If neurotransmitters inhibit a neuron, it does not fire or send on a signal. "The brain functions properly when there is a balance between the excitation and the inhibition. If there is either too much excitation or too little inhibition in a part of the brain (an imbalance), a seizure results," notes the American College of Physicians *Home Medical Guide.*[2]

When a seizure occurs, brain cells discharge rapidly— up to four times their normal rate. Some experts say this is like an electrical storm that may begin in one part of the brain and spread to other parts. Or the "storm" may originate on both sides of the brain at once.

STRUCTURE OF THE BRAIN

Because the nature of a seizure depends on where it originates in the brain, it's important to know something about the functions of different parts. The brain is divided into left and right hemispheres and each hemisphere has four lobes called the frontal, temporal, parietal (pu RI i tul), and occipital
(ok SIP i tl). Each of these lobes has different functions.

The frontal lobes affect movement, with the right frontal lobe involved in movement on a person's left side and just the opposite for the left frontal lobe. An injury to the left frontal lobe, for example, can cause motor impairment on the right side. The frontal lobes help produce speech and make decisions.

The functions of the temporal lobes are not as well understood as the other lobes, but they are responsible for distinguishing various sounds, tastes, and smells. They also help maintain balance and form memories. When temporal lobe seizures occur repeatedly over time, the *hippocampus* may be affected. The hippocampus is an area at the base of the brain that plays a role in one's memory and has been compared to the RAM of a computer. It stores data for a short time until it becomes part of the brain's long-term memory. The hippocampus can be damaged by repeated seizures.

Axons may be very short, such as those that carry signals from one cell in the cortex to another cell less than a hair's width away. Or axons may be very long, such as those that carry messages from the brain all the way down the spinal cord.

When the signal reaches the end of the axon it stimulates tiny sacs (5) that release chemicals known as neurotransmitters (6) into the synapse (7). The neurotransmitters cross the synapse and attach to receptors (8) on the neighboring cell. These receptors can change the properties of the receiving cell. If the receiving cell is also a neuron, the signal can continue the transmission to the next cell. (*Source: National Institute of Neurological Disorders and Stroke, Brain Basics: Know Your Brain* [Bethesda, Md.: Office of Communications, National Institutes of Health, 1992])

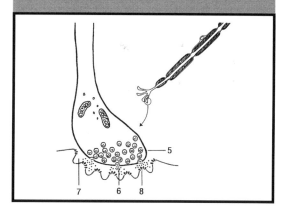

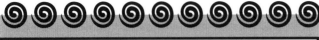

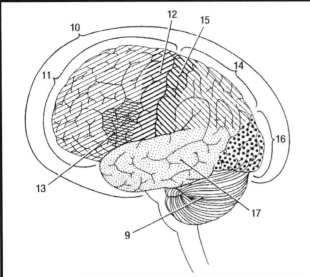

A wrinkled ball of tissue called the cerebellum (9) is part of the hindbrain, which controls the body's vital functions such as respiration and heart rate. The cerebrum (10) is part of the forebrain, the largest and most highly developed part of the human brain; it sits at the topmost part of the brain and is the source of intellectual activities and memories. The two frontal lobes (11) lie directly behind the forehead. At the rear of each frontal lobe is a motor area (12), which helps control voluntary movement. A nearby place on the left frontal lobe called Broca's area (13) allows thoughts to be transformed into words. The two sections behind the frontal lobes are called the parietal lobes (14), and the forward parts of these lobes, just behind the motor areas, are the primary sensory areas (15). At the back of the brain are the occipital lobes (16). The temporal lobes (17) nest under the parietal and frontal lobes. (*Source: National Institute of Neurological Disorders and Stroke, Brain Basics: Know Your Brain* [Bethesda, Md.: Office of Communications, National Institutes of Health, 1992])

Interpreting sensations (touch and spatial perception, for example) is the job of the parietal lobes, and the occipital lobes are involved in vision.

SEIZURES

If a person has a seizure, the event itself does not necessarily indicate that she or he has epilepsy. A seizure might occur, for example, because of a reaction to anesthesia or a strong medication. In some cases, children have seizures when they are ill with a high fever. Also, some people have what appear to be seizures but are events related to other medical conditions such as narcolepsy (sudden attacks of deep sleep) and Tourette's syndrome (facial or limb twitching and other involuntary behavior).

Only when a person has recurrent seizures is he or she considered to have epilepsy. Medical experts have identified more than thirty different types of seizures, but seizures are categorized by two main types: partial seizures and generalized seizures. Each of these two types is divided into subtypes.

A *partial seizure* originates in one part of the brain, an area that is known as the "focus." The National Institute of Neurological Disorders and

Stroke (NINDS) says that approximately "60 percent of people with epilepsy have partial seizures" and these are usually "described by the area of the brain in which they originate. For example, someone might be diagnosed with partial frontal lobe seizures."[3]

There are two common types of partial seizures: simple and complex. A *simple partial seizure* is usually short term, and a person is conscious and aware. If it's a temporal lobe seizure, symptoms may include smells that are not real (such as burning food, although no food is being cooked), unprovoked feelings of fear or anger, or a vivid memory.

Did you know? The human brain contains about 10 billion neurons, but the total number of neurons in a grasshopper's brain is only a few thousand.

In *complex partial seizures* a person's consciousness is usually altered, producing a dreamlike condition. People having complex partial seizures may stare blankly, twitch, fumble with clothing, make repetitive mouth movements, walk in circles, or display other *automatisms*—repetitious movements. A young woman whose partial seizures began when she was seventeen reported that "I always know when I'm about to have a seizure. All of a sudden I can't speak properly. . . . I know the word I want to say, but I just cannot say it. . . . As the seizure worsens I completely lose my ability to speak. I simply sit there in a dreamy world. I'm aware of what's happening around me, I just can't interact with my surroundings."[4]

There are various types of generalized seizures. One is called an *absence seizure*, also known as *petit mal*.

An absence seizure usually affects children, and a child may stare into space, become immobile, or have muscle spasms for a brief time—usually seconds. Parents, teachers, and other adults often misinterpret such behavior and may demand that a youngster "pay attention" or "stop daydreaming!" or "get with it!" But the child who experiences absence seizures is not aware of them and

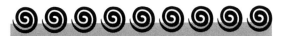

WHAT'S A BRAIN?

▶ It weighs less than 3 pounds (1.1 to 1.4 kg).
▶ It looks like a wrinkled walnut.
▶ It has the texture of thick jelly or gelatin.
▶ It's part of the central nervous system.
▶ It's what makes each person unique and is involved in emotions, thoughts, memory, sensations, dreams, and the control of movements.
▶ It's made up of billions of nerve cells called neurons.
▶ Its main parts are the right and left cerebral hemispheres and the brain stem.
▶ Its two hemispheres are connected in the middle.
▶ Its outer layer is gray matter made up of nerve cell bodies.
▶ Its inner layer is white matter comprised of insulated nerve fibers.
▶ It's like an electrical system that can receive and transmit messages.[5]

may have such spells hundreds of times during a day.

Generalized seizures also include tonic seizures, characterized by stiffening of the leg, arm, and back muscles, and clonic seizures that involve jerking of the muscles on both sides of the body. A *tonic-clonic* (or *grand mal*) *seizure* causes a mixture of symptoms. Neurons fire rapidly on both sides of the brain at about the same time. During the tonic phase of the seizure, all the body muscles may contract, making the body rigid and forcing air out of the lungs, which results in a high-pitched cry. A person loses consciousness, falling to the floor or ground and sometimes turning blue. During the clonic phase, the muscles contract, causing rhythmic jerking motions. Sometimes there is loss of bowel or bladder control. Falls due to tonic-clonic seizures can cause cuts, bruises, and other injuries.

A type of epileptic condition that can be life threatening is called *status epilepticus*. This refers to a prolonged seizure—one that lasts more than twenty minutes—or to a condition in which a person has one seizure after another without regaining consciousness. Emergency action is required.

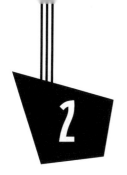

Fact or Folklore?

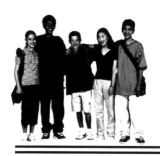

Throughout the ages, people have described epilepsy in hundreds of different ways, but little was really known about this brain disorder until the nineteenth century. According to the World Health Organization (WHO) an "ancient and detailed account of epilepsy is on a Babylonian tablet in the British Museum in London. This is a chapter from a Babylonian textbook of medicine comprising forty tablets dating as far back as 2000 B.C. The tablet accurately records many of the different seizure types we recognize today."

THE "SACRED DISEASE"

Babylonians were convinced that epilepsy was related to the supernatural and each type of seizure was named for a god or spirit. The ancient Greeks carried on this belief and associated epilepsy with the spiritual, calling it "the sacred disease." It was also believed that the moon god Selene was responsible for epilepsy, and people with epilepsy were thought to be "moonstruck," or "lunatics" (the Latin version of the word). Treatment ranged from eating mistletoe to drinking dog urine to purges and bloodletting. The idea was to rid the body of evil spirits.

During the fifth century B.C., the Greek medical scientist Hypocrites attempted to debunk beliefs about the spiritual nature of illnesses. In a collection of writings called the *Hippocratic Corpus,* Hypocrites and his followers argue against the idea that various diseases and disorders were caused by the gods. Hypocrites taught that epilepsy was a brain disorder, but his teachings did not dispel the widespread belief that people with epilepsy were demon-possessed.

Ancient Romans continued to believe in demon possession and thought epilepsy was contagious. Anyone who touched

While advances in technology enable film to create representations that are larger than life, many of the messages . . . [convey] harmful and dated information. One example is the portrayal of epilepsy. . . . To depict people with epilepsy as violent, crazed and frightening is inaccurate and destructive.

—Toba Schwaber Kerson, Professor of Social Work and Social Research, Bryn Mawr

9

someone with epilepsy, it was believed, could be taken over by an evil spirit. A variety of magical practices were thought to provide protection, such as bans on eating certain foods, wearing black clothing, and taking baths. Drinking human blood was also considered a protective measure—a way for a person with epilepsy to prevent a seizure.

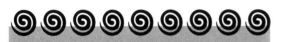

PHOTOSENSITIVE EPILEPSY

Photosensitive epilepsy is a condition in which moving or flickering lights can trigger a seizure. These flickering lights may come from such sources as computer monitors, video games, television, strobe lights, fluorescent tubes, and even sunlight reflecting on water.

Less than 5 percent of people with epilepsy today are photosensitive, and the frequency of flashing light that may provoke a seizure varies from person to person. Generally lights that flicker five to thirty times per second can trigger a seizure in photosensitive people.

How did ancient Romans determine whether people had epilepsy, or the "falling sickness" as it was called? The common practice was to have a suspected person smell a piece of jet. "If the person did not fall to the ground on smelling the stone, he was considered to be 'free of the falling sickness,'" according to the Epilepsy Museum in Germany. "A similar test was undertaken using a potter's wheel. It was believed that a person with epilepsy would fall to the ground on watching the wheel turn."[1] That turning wheel might have actually caused a seizure if a person was photosensitive. Today it is known that epileptic seizures can be triggered in photosensitive people by neon lights, flashing lights in discos, computer games, or certain television programs.

DRIVING OUT DEMONS

During the early Christian era, epilepsy was still considered the work of evil spirits who possessed individuals. This idea is clearly presented in the biblical book of Mark. According to the *New Living Translation*, the Apostle Mark tells of a man who brought his son to Jesus for a healing. The man explains that his son "can't speak because he is possessed by an evil spirit that won't let him talk. And whenever this evil spirit seizes him, it throws him violently to the ground and makes him foam at the mouth and grind his teeth and become rigid."

According to Mark, just as the boy was brought to Jesus, an evil spirit "threw the child into a violent convulsion, and he fell to the ground, writhing and foaming at the mouth." Jesus commanded the evil spirit to leave the child. "Then the spirit screamed and threw the boy into another violent convulsion and left him. The boy lay there motionless, and he appeared to be dead. . . . But Jesus took him by the hand and helped him to his feet, and he stood up."[2]

This biblical account, scholars say, describes a tonic-clonic seizure and the belief that an evil spirit had to be cast out by divine healing powers. Today it is an objective fact that anyone who has a tonic-clonic seizure usually suffers the symptoms presented in the biblical passage, can lose consciousness briefly, gradually revive, and be helped to sit or stand up.

In Europe during the Middle Ages, the idea of demon possession continued. But medieval Christians believed that prayers and sacred objects would protect against epilepsy or cure seizures. People fasted, made pilgrimages to sacred places, and called on saints, who were thought to have the power to intercede on behalf of someone with epilepsy. One of the most popular saints was Valentine of Germany. People seeking cures visited places where St. Valentine supposedly lived, and at one site in Alcase a hospital for epileptics was built during the fifteenth century. Since medieval times St. Valentine has been considered the patron saint of epilepsy.

For centuries, people with epilepsy not only suffered because of their disorder but also because of maltreatment by society at large. It was common to shun people who had seizures, isolating them in hospitals or other institutions because of fears that epilepsy was contagious. Punishment was another common treatment, especially when epilepsy was associated with witchcraft or the devil's work. Some people with epilepsy were thought to be witches and were burned at the stake.

Even royalty suffered brutal treatment. Consider King Charles II of England who had a seizure in 1685 while he was being shaved. At least a dozen physicians cared for him, but their treatments would hardly be called humane by today's standards. Doctors tried to purge his body by

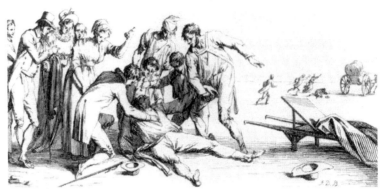

A nineteenth-century engraving shows a man suffering a seizure.
Source: The National Library of Medicine.

bloodletting, forcing him to vomit, administering enemas and laxatives repeatedly, and applying plasters made of pigeon dung to his feet. The king's head was also shaved so that blistering agents could be applied to his scalp. The king did not improve, so he was given concoctions that included numerous herbs, extracts from a human skull, and ammonia water. Nothing helped. King Charles II died within two days, no doubt due in part to his treatments.

MORE RECENT HISTORY OF EPILEPSY TREATMENT

During the eighteenth and early nineteenth centuries, epilepsy treatment began to change somewhat. Yet people who had frequent and/or prolonged epileptic seizures and could not be cared for by family members were sometimes institutionalized in prisons, in asylums for the mentally handicapped or insane, or in places that once housed people with leprosy. By the middle of the 1800s, a more humane concept developed and homes and hospitals for epileptic patients were opened in Europe.

In the 1800s, a London neurologist, John Hughlings Jackson, presented his theory that seizures were caused by "occasional, sudden, excessive, rapid, and local discharges of grey matter."[4] Dr. Jackson also found that particular parts of the brain control specific parts of the body. Thus, he concluded, the characteristics of a seizure depend on where discharges take place in the brain. Today one type of seizure, which begins with a twitch in the toe or thumb and spreads to the leg or arm, leading to a convulsion, is called the jacksonian "march" or jacksonian seizure.

Jackson's theories helped counteract the myth that epilepsy was a form of insanity and led to other theories and neurological discoveries. For example, in the 1920s Hans Berger, a German psychiatrist, developed the electroencephalograph (EEG), a test which reveals electrical discharges in the brain. The EEG confirmed the earlier Jackson assumptions and showed that the patterns of brainwave discharges vary with different types of seizures. With the EEG test, doctors were also able to locate where discharges originated.

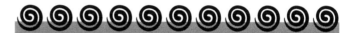

EPILEPSY "COLONIES"

According to the WHO:
A hospital for the "paralyzed and epileptic" was established in London in 1857. At the same time a more humanitarian approach to the social problems of epilepsy resulted in the establishment of epilepsy "colonies" for care and employment. Examples include Dianalund in Denmark, Chalfont in England, Bielefeld-Bethel in Germany, Heemstede in Holland, Sandviakain in Norway and the epilepsy centre in Zurich in Switzerland.[3]

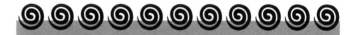

DEVELOPING ANTIEPILEPTIC DRUGS

Although animal models are used today to test new antiepileptic drugs, in the past such experiments did not take place. Doctors observed patients who were taking drugs for other purposes, noting that some of those medications could diminish seizures. During the 1850s, for example, Sir Charles Locock found that potassium bromide could help prevent seizures. He learned this because he was treating pregnant women and mistakenly believed that female epilepsy originated in the womb.

Bromides were used to treat epilepsy until 1912, when Dr. Alfred Hauptmann of Germany published the first paper on the use of luminal, now known as phenobarbitone. This was the beginning of a new era in effective treatment for epilepsy. But it was not until 1939 that two American doctors, H. Houston Merritt and Tracy J. Putnam, introduced phenytoin, which became the most effective medication for controlling seizures at that time.

Did you know? H. Houston Merritt, M.D. (1902–1979), is considered one of the greatest academic neurologists of the twentieth century. Under his leadership, the Neurological Institute of New York and Columbia-Presbyterian Medical Center achieved international recognition. Merritt with Tracy Putnam, M.D., discovered Dilantin, still a first-line drug for the treatment of epilepsy. The two doctors also established a scientific basis for identifying antiepileptic drugs and showed that an effective antiseizure medication did not have to be a sedative.

The first antiepileptic drugs were bromides, introduced in 1857 by Sir Charles Locock, an English physician. Locock found that sodium bromide, a sedative, reduced epileptic seizures. Other medications introduced in the early 1900s were phenobarbital and phenytoin, known by the trade name Dilantin. (Currently there are about two dozen drugs to treat seizures.)

In spite of advances in scientific knowledge and understanding of epilepsy, it was common in the United States during the 1920s and 1930s to bar people with epilepsy from public places and forbid them to marry. Sterilization laws in nearly half the states also required them to have an operation to prevent reproduction.

During the twentieth century numerous folk cures also were popular in treating epilepsy. Screen and TV star Danny Glover says his grandmother, who was convinced that someone had put a hex on him, insisted that he drink glass after glass of grape juice to cure his seizures. However, from the time he was first diagnosed with epilepsy at the

Did you know? One superstitious practice to ward off an epileptic seizure was to wear an amulet, or lucky charm, or to hang an amulet on a baby's cradle to prevent convulsions. Another practice from the past was to scrape matter from a human skull and give this to epileptic patients as a "cure." For a male patient, the matter had to come from a female skull and just the opposite for a female patient.

age of fifteen to age thirty-five when his seizures stopped, Glover controlled his epilepsy with Dilantin.[5]

WHAT CAUSES EPILEPSY AND SEIZURES?

As American and European medical experts became more enlightened about epilepsy, they continued to search for causes and treatment. That research is still under way today.

There are many possible causes for epileptic seizures. Anything that leads to an abnormal pattern of neuron activity, such as a brain injury at birth, a head injury due to a car accident, or a brain tumor, can cause epilepsy. Genes can play a role, with some people inheriting a predisposition for a gene disorder that leads to abnormal brain activity. Brain infections such as encephalitis and meningitis are responsible for some seizures, and people with AIDS, tuberculosis, or Jakob-Crutzfeldt disease may develop epilepsy. In the late stages of Alzheimer's, about one-third of those with this degenerative brain disease are likely to have seizures. Alcohol and other drug abuse can cause brain damage leading to epileptic seizures.

A variety of other medical problems such as diabetes (high levels of glucose or sugar in the blood due to lack of

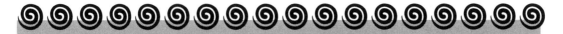

CORRECTING MYTHS & MISUNDERSTANDINGS

Q. Can a person inherit epilepsy?

A. Some rare forms of epilepsy are inherited, and some people might have a genetic makeup that leads to epileptic seizures. But most epilepsies are not inherited.

Q. Is epilepsy contagious?

A. Absolutely not.

Q. Is epilepsy a psychological problem?

A. No.

Q. Can epilepsy be cured?

A. Although there is no known cure for epilepsy, seizures in most people can be partially or fully controlled with treatment.

Q. Is epilepsy a lifelong condition?

A. Not necessarily. Many people with epilepsy do not have seizures throughout their entire lives.

Q. Does a person with epilepsy have "fits"?

A. A person with epilepsy experiences recurrent seizures; the outdated term "fits" suggests a person is hysterical or has gone mad—which is definitely not the case.

Q. Will a person with epilepsy become mentally retarded?

A. Epilepsy does not lead to mental retardation.

Q. Is epilepsy a mental or emotional illness?

A. No. It is a physical condition in which seizures are caused by excessive discharges of electricity in the brain.

Q. Can a person die from epilepsy?

A. Some people have seizures that are strong enough or prolonged enough to kill them. Others might have a fatal accident during a seizure, such as while climbing a high ladder or driving. But most people with epilepsy do not face life-threatening risks.

insulin) or hypoglycemia (low blood sugar) can cause seizures, but not necessarily the chronic seizures of epilepsy. Once the medical problem is corrected, the seizures stop.

While neurologists, especially *epileptologists* who specialize in epilepsy, can pinpoint the cause for the disorder in some people, they are unable to determine what provokes epilepsy in between 65 and 70 percent of the cases. The unknown factors leading to this brain disorder may contribute to the myths and prejudices surrounding epilepsy that persist to this day.

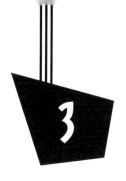

What's Happening?

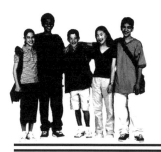

Many people with epilepsy, whether school-age or adult, cannot remember anything about the minutes or seconds before having a seizure. A seizure may happen when the person is asleep. Or there might be a sudden loss of consciousness. However, some people have *auras*, or unusual indicators before a seizure. These are described as a sour or bitter taste in the mouth, nausea, a "tight" feeling in the pit of the stomach, a tingling in the limbs, or an intense ringing in the ears. Such symptoms are "actually simple partial seizures in which the person maintains consciousness," according to the National Institute of Neurological Disorders and Stroke (NINDS).[1]

When I had my first seizure, I fell up against a [space] heater and burned myself pretty bad; no one knew what happened to me.

—Danny Glover, actor

Although individuals do not experience seizures in exactly the same way, those who can recall the onset of a seizure frequently relate common warning symptoms, such as these:

"I feel light-headed."

"I feel very depressed and can't relax."

"I am so tense I feel like I'm going to burst."

"People tell me I get a vacant look on my face."

"My hand starts to shake."

"A sense of extreme fear pervades, like I'm going to be killed but can't escape."

"I get confused as I try to say or write something."

"I feel very warm and begin to sweat."

"I can't concentrate."

PERSONAL STORIES

"When I was sixteen, classes started going by really fast. Not because the teachers were so fascinating, but because I couldn't seem to pay attention. . . . I couldn't make myself pay attention—the harder I tried, the worse it got. I would find myself in front of a classroom and not know what I was doing there (somebody in the class would let me know that I was in the middle of a speech)."[2]

These words by Christine Hagenlocher, posted on an Internet site, are the beginning of a long story about her frustrating struggle to find out what was happening to her and the problems she faced trying to convince her parents and medical professionals that she needed help. She was eventually diagnosed with epilepsy.

Sean

Sean's story also begins the year he was sixteen. A resident of the Washington, D.C., area, Sean is co-author of this book. He says his first seizure was in January 1985, six months after his sixteenth birthday:

The last thing I remember that Sunday morning was reading Hagar the Horrible *in the Sunday comics. The next thing I know I'm in a daze. I can tell by the sound that the front door is open and that a vehicle with power generators—which I correctly assume to be an ambulance—is outside. But I still can't focus my thoughts. I know I'm on the floor, very weak and that I can't get up.*

Finally, I hear someone say, "OK, he's coming around now. What's his name? ('Sean') Sean, do you know what day it is?"

"Saturday," I manage to mumble.

"OK, one day off."

I actually heard the paramedic say that. All this time, my mind is doing a continuous systems check. I can think, but I can't act.

Gradually my mind started to clear. I recognized where I was and what was happening. Somewhere in this, they told me I had had a seizure. I just sort of accepted that, not really knowing the implications in my current state of mind.

Because there are many reasons for seizures and epilepsy is only one of them, paramedics and other medical practitioners asked Sean numerous questions over the next few days. Had he had head injuries? Had he been diagnosed with chemical imbalances? Did he use illegal drugs—ever? An honest answer to this latter question is important, Sean emphasizes, because a truthful answer will aid in diagnosis. Fortunately, he could answer the question honestly. He had never used drugs.

After an overnight stay in the hospital, which included a lumbar puncture, or spinal tap, Sean learned that he had had a seizure, a *grand mal* seizure. "From my First Aid training in Boy Scouts, I knew what a seizure was—or thought I did," he says. "But I would soon discover that many misconceptions still exist about epileptic seizures." Sean was then referred to a pediatric neurologist. As he explains:

Pediatric neurologists handle patients up to age 17. I was 16 and a half. While I wasn't the oldest patient they had, I was considerably older than most of the other patients. Most of the chairs in the waiting area functioned better as footrests for me. And I found that reading literature in the waiting room was, oddly enough, medically oriented—written by some doctor named Seuss. I really couldn't understand why anyone would want to do a study on green eggs. Probably a federal grant.

I was quite fortunate to be assigned to a neurologist, Dr. John David Daigh, who was willing to talk frankly with me about my condition. He started me on the standard series of tests available at that time: blood work, computed tomography (CT) scan—a brain scan that shows the structure of the brain, and electroencephalo-grams (EEGs)—tests that record brain waves. We found that there actually was a brain inside my skull (a surprise to some); and that it did function, if not quite properly.

Sean's EEG showed an irregularity, but it wasn't conclusive. However, he soon learned that he suffered from tonic-clonic seizures. Nevertheless, as Sean put it, "they didn't know why I was having grand mal seizures." To this day, no one has been able to figure out why his seizures occur, which is a complication, "but it doesn't make the disorder any more severe in reality," he says.

Alyssa

On a ThinkQuest Internet site, Alyssa, now a teenager, tells how she discovered in 1996, when she was in elementary school, that she had epilepsy. She woke up one morning on the floor, feeling

incredibly sick, and the light bothered my eyes. I shut every light in the house off. I couldn't see very well, either, everything looked wavy, like if you need glasses and you go to the bathroom in the middle of the night without your glasses. The funny thing was, I don't need glasses. My Mom called my Dad to come home from work to take care of my brother, and took me to the hospital. I couldn't stop throwing up, even in the car. Luckily, I had a strong plastic bag with me.

When I got to the hospital, I got a whole bunch of tests. First they took a blood test, to see if I had swallowed any poison. Then about 6 different doctors examined me. They all thought I was a perfectly healthy kid, with nothing wrong. They couldn't figure anything out. Then I got a CAT scan to see if I had a head injury or brain tumor. The CAT scan machine is a narrow white tube, and you lay down in it and can't move. The test only goes on for a few minutes. The CAT scan machine takes X-rays of little slices of your brain. It uses just a little radiation, so it doesn't damage your brain. Everyone else has to leave the room while the machine is taking the X-rays. Since I was so little, the technician let me take my stuffed fox into the CAT scan machine with me. The technicians and my Mom could talk to me through a microphone from the glass control booth. It was kind of fun. Then they wheeled me back to the emergency room in a wheelchair, even though by then I felt fine.

Everyone kept talking about my seizure. I didn't know what "seizure" meant. The doctors told my mom that I probably had a seizure because my blood sugar was low, but that she should bring me back for an EEG just to be sure.

I went back to the hospital and had an EEG. That's when they paste these little wires to your head and attach them to a machine to measure your brain waves. The technician measured my head, and marked my scalp with a grease pencil. Then she scrubbed the spots she marked with an itchy, rough paste so the wires would stick. Then she stuck the wires to my head with big gobs of paste. It was very boring, and the paste was very itchy, and it was impossible to get out of my hair.

My brain waves were abnormal. That's how they found out I had epilepsy. I was pretty scared when I first found out that I had epilepsy. My first question was could I still be a field biologist when I grow up, which was what I've wanted to do since I was three. My mom told me "of course you can." When I heard that, I felt much more relieved.[3]

Dania

Dania's story, written when she was seventeen years old, notes that she'd had one convulsive seizure when she was fourteen, but numerous *petit mal* (absence) seizures

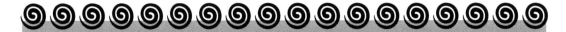

TEEN SUPPORT GROUPS

Adolescents with epilepsy who find it difficult to openly discuss their disorder often can find help through support groups. Some support groups can be accessed on the Internet where chat rooms offer people with epilepsy an opportunity to ask questions, share information, and "talk" informally with one another. Other support groups form so that people can meet face-to-face and share their concerns.

Numerous support groups that cater to teens with epilepsy have formed across the country. Such groups are initiated by affiliates of the Epilepsy Foundation, hospitals, religious organizations, or by individual teens. For example, Kristen Pollock of Seneca, South Carolina, a high school senior who has epilepsy, started a teen epilepsy support group at her school to provide peer support to others with epilepsy and raise awareness of the disorder. She was named a top student volunteer and given the Prudential Spirit of Community Award in 2001. In addition South Carolina honored her with a resolution (Senate Bill 370) congratulating her on her "outstanding record of volunteer service, peer leadership and community spirit."

Most teen support groups include no more than a dozen young people with a facilitator, or group leader. The facilitator is usually a health care professional, social worker, or other person knowledgeable about epilepsy and the psychological and social concerns facing teens with epilepsy. Such a person is able to correct erroneous information about epilepsy and lead group discussions. Topics frequently discussed are overprotective parents, employment, sexuality, dating, driving, and explaining seizures to classmates, teachers, and others.

Within a support group, adolescents can learn to speak freely and develop social skills and self-confidence. Teens in support groups also learn how to deal with other's prejudices about epilepsy and how to counteract misconceptions with facts.

before and after that time. Here's how she described her experience:

> I have always hated being different and having to take pills and getting tired from pills as my body got used to dosage increases or decreases. I told all of my friends, and am not embarrassed, but just wish it would go away. This year especially has been tough. Since I am not labeled as epileptic, I am allowed to have my license, but my mom is still very scared about me getting into an accident since on rare occasions, I do get petit mals.
>
> We argue a lot about this, because I want to be a "normal" teenager. This year, I decided to do my focus

project on children and teenagers who suffer from epilepsy. This has really helped me come to terms with my differences, and I feel a lot better hearing other similar stories. I have learned that you can make it through this, and that it isn't that bad, just be strong.[4]

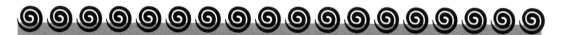

TAKEDOWN (A TEEN NOVEL)

In times past, writers such as Shakespeare, Fyodor Dostoyevski, and Charles Dickens created characters who had epilepsy. But such characters appear in only a few modern-day novels. An example is the teenage novel, *Takedown* by E. M. J. Benjamin, a pen name for a two-person writing team, one of them a high school wrestling coach.

In the story, seventeen-year-old Jake is the central character, a high-school wrestler whose coach constantly drills the team on takedowns. "Think how important the takedown is . . . it's that critical moment when you get the other guy off balance and take him to the mat," the coach tells them. Jake may complain about practice, but he's dedicated to winning the high school wrestling title.

After several seizures, which are preceded by auras, a "rotten-cheese smell," as Jake describes it, he learns he has epilepsy. His reaction mirrors many real-life cases of young people who receive this diagnosis. Members of Jake's family, Chopper, a younger brother, and his parents, also react in a typical fashion. However, Chopper, a computer whiz, has searched the Internet for information on seizures, sharing his knowledge with Jake, who doesn't really want to believe what his brother tells him.

The story realistically portrays Jake's attempts to deal with epilepsy. At first he is in denial, then he's angry and asks the "why me?" question in a variety of different ways. Jake decides not to tell anyone he has epilepsy—not his friends, not his coach. He calls himself "The Great Liar" and uses numerous subterfuges to keep from revealing his disorder. Jake also has to deal with taking his medication daily and, as happens in real life, he sometimes forgets, triggering a seizure one evening while out of town for a wrestling meet.

Jake can no longer hide his condition, but he withdraws. His coach, friends, and his father try to bring Jake back. Eventually he does stop "cocooning"—feeling sorry for himself—and comes to terms with epilepsy. He gains control of his life.

(*Source:* E. M. J. Benjamin, *Takedown* [Wilmington, N.C.: Banks Channel Books, 1999]).

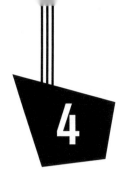

4 Diagnosis and Treatment

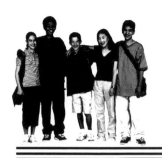

People who have experienced epileptic seizures often describe how they were first diagnosed with epilepsy and also what kind of treatment was prescribed. After a first seizure, however, a correct diagnosis is not necessarily a simple matter. As two British physicians explained in their book on epilepsy: "There are three possible preliminary diagnoses"—first, the patient had a seizure; second, the person had some kind of attack or blackout but *not* a seizure; and third, the person may have had a seizure but it's not certain. Then a doctor has to decide whether to continue with an investigation. Finally, choices must be made about whether to prescribe treatment or wait to see if other seizures occur. In brief, the medical decisions about what course to take can be complex.[1]

By far the most common approach to treating epilepsy is to prescribe antiepileptic drugs.

—National Institute of Neurological Disorders and Stroke, National Institutes of Health

COLLECTING INFORMATION

One of the first tools in diagnosing epilepsy is collecting accurate information about what a patient felt and was doing before and after losing consciousness. Obviously someone who is unconscious cannot provide any of the details, but an eyewitness may be able to give a doctor important information. That eyewitness is likely to be a parent, friend, classmate, teacher, co-worker—or perhaps even a stranger.

What types of questions do doctors ask observers? Some examples:

When did the event (seizure) take place?

Were there any warning signs that the person was losing consciousness?

How long was the person unconscious?

How did the person act during and after the seizure?

A doctor will also ask the patient such questions as: Do you use drugs or have a history of alcohol abuse? Have you had any head injuries? Have you had meningitis? There will also be questions about the family history: Do other family members have epilepsy? Were there any problems at birth?

After clinical information is gathered, a doctor may order a thorough neurological examination, which commonly includes an EEG.

THE EEG

The EEG is a valuable and painless test in diagnosing epilepsy. It can be administered while the patient is awake

Qs & As ABOUT EEGs

Q. Does an EEG cause an electrical shock?

A. No. The procedure is painless.

Q. Does the gel used to attach electrodes damage the hair?

A. No. The gel can be washed out.

Q. What makes the pens move during an EEG?

A. Electrodes pick up the tiny electrical charges in the brain and the electroencephalograph amplifies these charges, sending them to the series of pens. Electrical activity makes the pens move.

Q. Is an EEG considered a treatment for epilepsy?

A. No. It is a test to obtain information about the brain's electrical activity.

Q. Where are EEG tests given?

A. Usually in a clinic or outpatient facility connected with a hospital.

or asleep. The normal waking EEG detects and records the brain's electrical patterns—brain waves. How does it work?

About two dozen small disks called electrodes are attached with a gel to various locations on the head. Wires from the disks are connected to an electroencephalograph, a machine that records the brain's electrical patterns and stores them on a computer or prints out the brain waves on paper.

A patient has to lie quietly during an EEG test, because body movements could alter the results. But the technician administering the test, which lasts from sixty to ninety minutes, asks a patient to perform several actions that can stimulate brain waves, such as breathing rapidly, opening and closing the eyes, and looking at flashing lights.

A neurologist who analyzes an EEG will distinguish between what is normal and abnormal in a person's brain waves. "When a person is healthy, the electrical messages to and from the brain tend to produce characteristic patterns of *alpha waves* and *beta waves*," according to Canadian Professor of Neurology Donald Weaver. "Alpha waves normally appear when the person is awake and

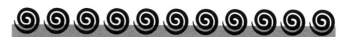

LEFTY CARMICHAEL HAS A FIT (A TEEN NOVEL)

The offbeat but realistic characters in this teenage novel have little or no knowledge about epilepsy at the beginning of this story, which is set in a tough, working-class neighborhood. Teenage and adult characters frequently use an outdated term (*fit*) to describe what happens when Lefty Charmichael has tonic-clonic seizures. In the novel, by Canadian author Don Trembath, Lefty has to come to grips with epilepsy and cope with friends and classmates who don't understand and fear his seizures, which are accurately portrayed along with the kind of treatment required.

However, the story itself is more than a medical discourse on epilepsy. It focuses on Lefty's relationships with his family, classmates, girlfriend, Penny, and best friend, Rueben. Although Lefty tries to handle his epilepsy with self-assurance, he has fights with classmates, is suspended from school, and becomes estranged from Penny and Reuben, eventually withdrawing from everyone. Penny grows impatient and irritated with Lefty and scolds him for letting "your seizures take over your life. You've stopped doing things. You've stopped having fun. All you do is read about epilepsy and write in your little notepad."

Lefty's struggle to take back his life makes up the final chapters of the book and includes a reconciliation with his friends. (*Source:* Don Trembath, *Lefty Charmichael Has a Fit* [Custer, Wash.: Orca Book Publishers, 1999]).

relaxed, with eyes closed. Beta waves appear when the person is awake but is slightly tense. Certain medications . . . may accentuate beta waves." Dr. Weaver explains that a person with epilepsy may have abnormal wave patterns known as *spikes, sharp waves,* and *spike waves.*[2]

However, an EEG is not flawless; it may not show an abnormal pattern even though a person has epilepsy. About 20 percent of people with epilepsy have a normal EEG. Between 2 and 5 percent of people who do *not* have epilepsy have abnormal changes on their EEG.

When there is uncertainty about a patient's condition, a doctor may have a patient wear or carry a portable EEG device to record brain waves over a twenty-four- or forty-eight-hour period. Video monitoring along with an EEG test during a seizure might also be ordered. In some cases, this requires that a person be deprived of sleep, which could initiate a seizure; a video camera then records a patient's activity during an EEG.

A patient may have to go to an Epilepsy Monitoring Unit (EMU) in the hospital for another type of video monitoring. The stay in an EMU ranges from several days to two weeks. What happens during this time? Doctors may instruct patients taking antiseizure drugs to decrease their dosages or discontinue their medications so that seizures can occur. Because patients are constantly wired to video and EEG monitoring equipment, they are not able to move around much, spending most of the time sitting in a bed or a chair. Electrodes stay on the head during the entire monitoring period, so patients can't wash their hair or take showers.

OTHER DIAGNOSTIC TOOLS

Along with EEGs, other important tools in diagnosing epilepsy are brain scans. The most frequently used scans include computed tomography (CT) and magnetic resonance imaging (MRI). CT and MRI scans show the brain's structure, helping a doctor identify abnormalities such as cysts and tumors.

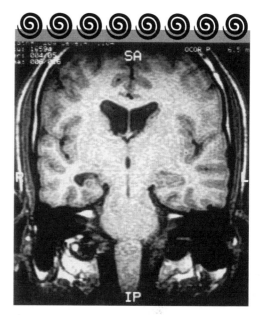

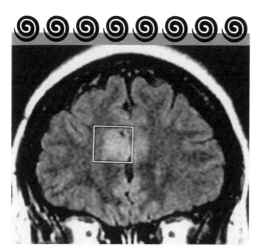

This MRI shows an abnormal formation in the frontal lobe, which is the cause of some epilepsies. *Courtesy of Susan Spencer, M.D., Department of Neurology, Yale University School of Medicine.*

This MRI scan shows an irregularity between the left and right sides of the hippocampus. This is a part of the temporal lobe that often is the area where uncontrolled seizures arise. (The left side of the image shows the right side of the brain—there is an R on that side.) There you can see the small hippocampus compared to the left side. *Courtesy of Susan Spencer, M.D., Department of Neurology, Yale University School of Medicine.*

MRIs are gradually replacing CT scans because the MRI scans produce more detailed images of the brain. If a teenager (or any other patient) is having one of these tests, she or he lies on a scanning table that slides into a tunnel-like machine. CT scans use X-rays; MRI scans do not. When an MRI scan is performed, a magnetic field is created and radio waves are beamed at the brain. Small particles called protons within the brain's atoms produce radio waves that are picked up and measured by a sensitive device and then analyzed by a computer that creates detailed pictures of the brain. "MRI can detect many subtle and small abnormalities that were previously undetectable by CT scanning. . . . MRI is especially useful in assessing the suitability of surgical treatment for patients who have not responded to drugs," according to the American College of Physicians.[3]

TREATMENT

If a person is diagnosed with epilepsy, what happens next? The most common treatment for epilepsy is daily use of anticonvulsant drugs. The oldest drugs are phenobarbital and Dilantin (phenytoin).

Altogether the United States Food and Drug Administration (FDA) has approved nearly two dozen different drugs for epilepsy treatment. Drugs have both trade names, which are capitalized, and generic names. They include Felbatol (felbamate), Neurontin (gabapentin), Lamictal (lamotrigine), Topamax (topiramate), Gabitril (tiagabine), Tegretol (carbamazepine), Depakote (Divalproex sodium), Keppra (levetiracetam), and Zonagran (zonisamide). In addition, FDA also has approved Diastat for at-home use. Diastat is used in emergency rooms to break a chain of seizures, which can be fatal if not stopped. Diastat is taken rectally and reaches the bloodstream in about two minutes.

How does a doctor determine which medication to prescribe? It depends on the kind of seizure a person is having. Drugs are designed to control different types of seizures.

When Sean first started having seizures, he took Depakote, a standard procedure for his type of epilepsy, but he had another seizure.

My dosage was increased, but I still had another seizure. My doctor then switched me to Tegretol. That appeared to be working, but one day I noticed some spots on my arm. At my next appointment, I learned that I was allergic to Tegretol and was switched to Dilantin. I had a few more seizures after that, but once the dosage was increased, I stopped having seizures—for a while.

Different people require different dosages of Dilantin or other medication. Because of the way people's bodies metabolize (process) medicine, the resulting amount left in the bloodstream, or level, can vary. Blood levels are measured in micrograms per milliliter, µg/ml. Therapeutic, or effective, levels of Dilantin, for example, are normally between ten and twenty. Some people can take a low dose and get a therapeutic level; for others, the reverse is true.

People with epilepsy may have to adjust their medications often in order to control their seizures. Even though a medication level may be in the therapeutic range, dosages may have to be increased or reduced slightly, or a person might have to switch from, say, Dilantin to phenobarbital. Or perhaps a combination of drugs is prescribed.

Whatever the course of therapy, it is important to learn about any medication, know what the right dosage is, how to take it, and what level is therapeutic. This information can be helpful if a person with epilepsy changes doctors due to a move or to requirements of a health insurance company. Sean explains that after several years dealing with his epilepsy, he became familiar with how his prescribed dosages of Dilantin worked for him. But he moved to a new location and started to have seizures again. He had to find a new neurologist, who was at a loss to explain why Dilantin had apparently stopped working. "She even accused me of lying to her about taking my medication," Sean says, adding:

If I have learned anything since my first seizure, it is that I must be totally honest with my doctor and thereby generate trust. One of the most difficult problems you face after a while is having to disagree with a doctor. During one such transition, a doctor who had been treating me for less than six months told me that I needed to reduce my Dilantin dosage. Because I had had epilepsy for fifteen years and had been seizure free for close to a year, I knew I needed a high therapeutic level of medication in order to be OK. But the doctor was worried about my liver. I should have known better. I started to have seizures again. Fortunately, I was able to get my old neurologist back.

THE KETOGENIC DIET

A controversial treatment for some young people with a severe form of epilepsy, especially those with intractable epilepsy, is the ketogenic diet. The modern form of this diet, which was introduced in the 1920s before antiseizure medications were widely available, is high in fats (such as vegetable oils and cream) and low in carbohydrates and protein. Carbohydrates are made up of sugars (glucose), and if they are decreased in the diet and fat is substituted instead, the body has no glucose source. For survival, the body breaks down fats instead of carbohydrates for fuel, producing a condition in the body known as ketosis. Ketosis "has been recognized since biblical times as beneficial for seizure control," writes Dr. Donald Weaver.[5] The condition was observed in people who had fasted or been on a near-starvation diet in order to reduce seizures.

There are numerous drawbacks to this diet, however. First and foremost, it is difficult to maintain and requires eating a limited number of fatty foods. Food and liquid intake must be carefully calculated and monitored each day. Even the amount of sugar in a pill must be counted. Side effects from the diet can include nausea, stomach cramps, and nutritional deficiencies that inhibit growth. Health care professionals caution that the diet should not be attempted without the guidance of a nutritionist or dietician.

Sean's medications were changed several times and one of the newer drugs, gabapentin, was added. But, he said, "My mind was really affected. It got to the point where my boss noticed, so I stopped taking my medication altogether, without telling my doctor. NOT SMART—I DON'T RECOMMEND THIS." He eventually told his doctor and got back on track with his medications.

COMBATING SIDE EFFECTS

Noticeable side effects of some drug treatments for epilepsy are lack of energy or drive and the inability to concentrate. Overcoming the side effects of anticonvulsants may be possible with another medication known as Ritalin, commonly used by patients who have attention deficit disorder.

Dr. J. Layne Moore, director of the comprehensive epilepsy program at the Ohio State University Medical Center, conducted a small pilot study and found that methylphenidate, marketed as Ritalin, helps to relieve some of the negative side effects of antiseizure medication, such as the inability to concentrate, slow mental function, and drowsiness. Still, Dr. Moore cautions that more studies need to be conducted to understand the role of methylphenidate in treating people with epilepsy.[4]

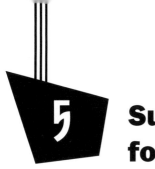

5 Surgery for Epilepsy

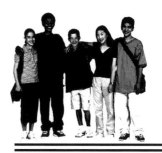

In some cases, medication does little to control seizures, and brain surgery may be considered. Any surgery carries risks, and certainly brain surgery is a major undertaking. But the decision to treat epilepsy with surgery is only made after a detailed assessment of a patient. This involves a team of neurologists, neurosurgeons, social workers, and perhaps psychiatrists. These specialists carefully evaluate such factors as the frequency and severity of seizures, the risk of brain damage from frequent seizures, as well as what economic and social impact surgery would have on a person's family and quality of life.

Patients who are candidates for brain surgery undergo numerous tests and are monitored intensively. The first test would likely be an electroencephalogram (EEG). An MRI (brain scan) would be performed to determine whether there are abnormalities such as tumors or scars that can prompt seizures. To locate the exact focus of seizures, doctors might implant electrodes into the brain or lay them on the surface of the brain to record brain activity, providing more information than is possible to obtain with an EEG. A test might be given in which the drug amobarbitol is injected to locate areas of the brain controlling memory and speech. Surgeons would need such information to avoid operating on that part of the brain.

Psychiatric testing may also be done for some patients. A psychiatric assessment helps rule out a mental illness, such as severe depression, that would prevent surgery until the illness could be successfully treated.

Many people [with epilepsy] who could benefit from surgery are not being referred for surgery because many doctors, insurance carriers and patients alike are unaware of this option for those whose seizures are not controlled by medications.

—UCLA Epilepsy Program

SUCCESS STORIES

Teenager Sean Merrill of Clarksville, Tennessee, was suffering an average of six epileptic seizures each day. In April 2000, he had surgery at Vanderbilt University Medical Center in Nashville, Tennessee, to remove about one-third of his brain. Neurosurgeons removed the areas where his seizures were originating—the left temporal lobe and a portion of the left hemisphere, which usually controls muscle movement on the right side. Surgery also included cutting nerve connections between the two halves of the brain so that seizures would not spread.

According to his surgeons, tests showed that the functions of the left side of Merrill's brain had been transferred to the right side and "the left side was doing very little for him except generating seizures."[1] During the eight-hour operation, surgeons "didn't use scalpels, but used the heated ends of a tweezer-like instrument to 'melt' the edges of the seizure-producing brain tissue so it could be gently removed with minimum damage to surrounding areas." About twenty-four hours after his operation, Sean Merrill "was able to sit up, speak and wiggle his feet. . . . That showed Sean's brain . . . had begun to heal."[2]

Kristen in Maryland had her first surgery for epilepsy when she was fifteen years old, but not all of the damaged area of her brain was removed. So five years later she had a second operation to remove her right temporal lobe and occipital lobe. She explained that before the second surgery, she could never go anywhere alone, not even for a walk outdoors. But now "finally I can, no more babysitting me! The meds are slowly being reduced and then maybe I can begin to think more clearly and relearn some of the things I have forgotten," she wrote.[3]

Until he had brain surgery, Texan Luke Potts had violent seizures that often left him cut and bruised. In high school he told his classmates that his injuries were due to sports—he didn't want anyone to know he had seizures, which began after he suffered a head injury as a youngster. The seizures intensified as he got older.

In 1996 at age sixteen, Luke's doctor recommended surgery, so the teenager finally
informed his friends about his disorder. They
rallied around, even shaving his head before
he went to the hospital in Houston. In an ex-
ploratory operation, doctors found that the
damaged area in his brain was "too close to
his speech center to remove it. So, they performed a subpial transection, surgically
scraping the brain's surface in hopes of re-
moving damaged tissue. It worked. Luke's
seizures were milder and 80 to 90 percent
less frequent, and his medication dosage de-
clined by two-thirds." Later on Luke had a
vagus nerve stimulator implanted to keep
him seizure free.[4]

Kristin Austin, a sixteen-year-old in Al-
berta, Canada, also reported successful brain
surgery to prevent seizures. She was diagnosed with epilepsy when she was eleven
years old and says her sixth-grade teacher
"actually was the one who picked up on the
fact that I was having seizures." An MRI revealed she had a deformity—a small benign
tumor—on the right side of her brain in the temporal lobe.
Her doctors recommended drug therapy to control the
seizures, but none of the
medications worked for
long. "I reached the
point where one
month all I did
was have a
seizure every day
and missed school
completely." In July
2001, she had sur-
gery to remove the tu-
mor (gangliocytoma)
that had a calcified area

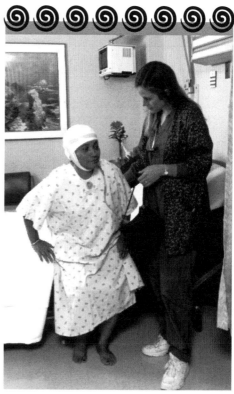

A patient is being monitored after brain
surgery. *Photo courtesy of Jerome Engel
Jr., M.D., Ph.D., Director Seizure Disorders Center, UCLA School of Medicine.*

Did you know? The cost of surgery
for epilepsy can range from $35,000 to
$150,000, depending on what type of
procedures are required. Total epilepsy
costs in the United States each year
are about $12.5 billion, which include
direct medical and related expenses
and indirect costs such as lost income.

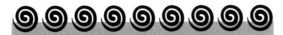

SEIZURE FREE

In her book *Seizure Free*, Leanne Chilton describes her experiences leading up to brain surgery, which included the EEG with video monitoring, an MRI, a CT scan, and neuropsychological testing. She learned that her numerous seizures were originating from the right side of her brain and that the right hippocampus and the right side of her temporal lobe would need to be removed. She writes:

It sounds scary when you put it down on paper, doesn't it? But if you are having seizures and your medication keeps you intoxicated most of the time, the word "surgery" sounds more like a miracle cure. Getting a part of your brain removed doesn't sound nearly as bad as living with seizures the rest of your life and being on medication that doesn't work too well. So if you are considering surgery for yourself or someone you know, this is the point where I have to tell you to hang in there.[6]

the size of a golf ball. Now she reports: "I am on the cheerleading squad at my school, learning tumbling, and a very active and healthy person." She is delighted that she has overcome "powerful odds, and am living like I wanted to for so long—normally like a teenager."[5]

TYPES OF SURGERY

The most common type of epilepsy surgery is *temporal lobe resection*, which involves removal of a portion of the temporal lobe where a seizure originates. Such surgery can reduce or halt seizures in people with temporal lobe epilepsy. A study conducted at University of Western Ontario in London found that "brain surgery virtually eliminated seizures in 58 percent of patients with temporal lobe epilepsy," according to a report in the *Journal of the American Medical Association*. Some epilepsy centers report that 80 percent or more of their patients with temporal lobe epilepsy are seizure free after surgery.[7]

Sometimes the focus of a seizure is in a part of the brain that cannot be removed. In such cases, surgeons might perform *multiple subpial transection*. Surgeons find the focus of seizures and try to separate that area from other parts of the brain by cutting nerve fibers to prevent a seizure from spreading. At the same time, normal functions of the brain are preserved.

People who have severe seizures that start in one hemisphere and spread to the other half of the brain may be helped with a surgical procedure called *corpus callosotomy*. A band of tissue called the corpus callosum between the two sides of the brain conducts electricity and passes mes-

sages. If the nerve connections between the two halves are cut, severe seizures may stop. However,
as the NINDS cautions, "the procedure does not stop seizures in
the side of the brain where they
originate, and these partial seizures
may even increase after surgery."[8]

VAGUS NERVE STIMULATOR

A fairly new type of surgical treatment for epilepsy involves the implant of device known as the
vagus nerve stimulator (VNS), approved in 1997 by the Food and
Drug Administration (FDA). The
device is rather like a pacemaker
for the heart and it is surgically

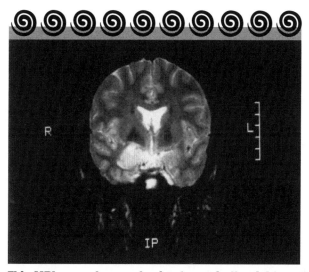

This MRI scan shows a benign tumor in the right temporal lobe, which is another cause of temporal lobe seizures. *Courtesy of Susan Spencer, M.D., Department of Neurology, Yale University School of Medicine.*

implanted under the skin. That is, a surgeon performs an
operation, making an incision in the chest to form a
"pocket" for a small VNS battery-operated pulse generator
attached to electrodes. A thin tube with electrodes is
threaded under the skin to another incision on the neck
where the vagus nerve is located. The tube is wrapped
around the vagus nerve, and after surgery, the pulse generator is set to automatically stimulate the vagus nerve at regular intervals. This sends electrical signals to the brain,
changes brain chemicals, and in most cases curbs seizures.

A doctor monitors a VNS implant every two weeks at
first and then every two to six months. With the use of a
computer and software the doctor can adjust the device's
rate of stimulation if needed.

Some people with VNS implants use a special magnet,
passing it over the chest area where the device is implanted,
to provide extra stimulation. For people who have an aura
or warning that a seizure is about to take place, use of the
magnet may stop a seizure or make it less severe.

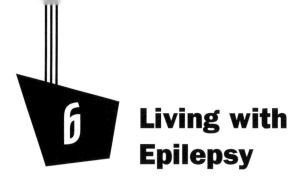

6 Living with Epilepsy

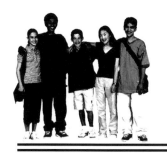

Maurizio Passero, who describes himself as an Italian Canadian, at the age of eleven had a brain aneurysm—a ruptured blood vessel in his brain—which left him paralyzed on the left side. "After the stroke I was put on the anticonvulsant drug Tegretol," Passero writes, "and I took my pills for a year without incident." Then he had his first seizure—"a big grand mal (tonic-clonic) seizure, which lasted about fifteen minutes. I was twelve years old."

Between the ages of twelve and sixteen, Passero had three more tonic-clonic seizures and also "a lot of auras—simple partial seizures—at night." At the time he didn't know the auras were seizures and neither did his parents. "I would run into their bedroom overcome with fear, or with the feeling I was going to throw up. Sometimes I was unresponsive when they asked me questions. I was considered to be acting like a baby." Passero explained that "In my culture, the emphasis is on strength—physical strength, mental toughness. It's considered bad to be weak." In addition, "the cultural belief is that if you have epilepsy or any kind of disability, you won't accomplish very much. Academically, no one expects anything of you. No one ever said to me: 'I can see you becoming great.' This is disempowering to people who have disabilities." He writes:

> My parents didn't push me at all in high school, and I took advantage of that and didn't work very hard. But then I spent a year . . . working construction in the winter and decided that I had to go back to school and make something of myself. I went to college, then to university to study social work.

People with controlled epilepsy are limited more often by public misperceptions and stereotypes than by the disorder itself.

—Steven Schachter, M.D., director of Clinical Research at the Comprehensive Epilepsy Center, Beth Israel Hospital, Boston, Massachusetts

School wasn't easy for me. Learning disorders from the stroke meant I had to work much harder than anybody else. It would take me twenty hours to finish something that my classmates could complete in two. . . . I have made it my mission to educate people—be it about epilepsy, racism, or any topic [about which] there is a lot of ignorance. I also want to help people. . . . Bringing epilepsy out of the shadows is very important. People need to be educated about seizure disorders, just like I did, in order to understand. There is a lot of ignorance out there.

Recently my dad said, "After what you've been through in your life, it's unbelievable what you've become." People with disabilities need a positive belief system. They need others who can envision them doing great things to tell them: "You can do anything you put your mind to."[1]

A TV CHARACTER WITH EPILEPSY

During the fall TV season in 2000, the police-action series *Nash Bridges* introduced a new character, black detective Antwon Babcock, played by actor Cress Williams. Babcock was presented as a detective who had been transferred from one police department to another, creating the perception that he was a troublemaker. But it was soon revealed that he had epilepsy, a historic first for a character appearing regularly in a TV series.

In a spring 2001 episode, Babcock went with a group of officers who broke into a warehouse that was rigged with strobe lights, blinding the officers. Babcock quickly announced: "I gotta get out of here." His reaction would be expected for someone whose seizures are triggered because of photosensitivity.

The show's fans had conflicting opinions about the way seizures were portrayed, however. One viewer who had witnessed her husband's seizures thought the depiction was "all wrong" because of the way the actor fell and because he was up and about in a few minutes. Some fans declared they knew little about epilepsy but were pleased to see a character with epilepsy included in the show. *Nash Bridges* is no longer aired, but reruns appear regularly.

EPILEPSY AND DRIVING

What teenager does *not* want to drive a car? Getting a driver's license is like a rite of passage, moving from one stage of life to another. Being able to drive provides a sense of freedom and independence. While teenagers whose seizures are controlled can drive safely and legally, the privilege of driving carries restrictions for some people who have epilepsy.

DRIVING RESTRICTIONS

Nearly all states require individuals with epilepsy to be seizure free for a certain time period before being allowed to drive. That time period can range from a few months to two years.

In Florida, for example, applicants and licensed drivers must be seizure free for a period of two years before being approved for licensing. In New Mexico, the seizure-free interval is usually one year. North Carolina requires a six- to twelve-month seizure-free period. Oklahoma's law requires just six months without having a seizure before a driver's license can be granted.

Only six states (California, Delaware, Nevada, New Jersey, Oregon, and Pennsylvania) mandate that doctors report someone they've diagnosed with epilepsy to the Department of Motor Vehicles, Department of Public Safety, Health Department, or other state agency. In California, for example, doctors must immediately report to the local health officer individuals whom they have diagnosed as having "a disorder characterized by lapses of consciousness."

In some states, laws require doctors to tell their patients with epilepsy not to drive, or risk being liable for accidents such patients cause. If patients ignore this medical advice, they are legally responsible for accidents even though no seizure is involved or even though they are not at fault.

In some states a person with epilepsy may be able to get a driver's license that carries restrictions such as daytime driving only. Or the license might be issued but limited to driving to and from work or only in an emergency. Once the person is seizure free for the state's specified time, the restrictions no longer apply.

Driver's licensing laws by state can be accessed via the Epilepsy Foundation web site http://www.epilepsyfoundation.org/answerplace/drivelaw/searchform.cfm.

In some cases, teenagers (and adults) continue to drive regardless of the risk of having seizures while on the road. Not surprisingly when seizures occur, accidents happen, sometimes causing property damage and injuries to those with epilepsy as well as others. Drivers have to determine whether peoples' lives (including their own) are at risk if they blank out or have a convulsion while behind the wheel.

Pamela is one young person who knows the inconvenience of these restrictions. She has had seizures since infancy but didn't learn she had epilepsy until she was in eighth grade. Her seizures continued through high school and her first year of college. She explained that she does not have convulsions. "I just black out and do weird things like take a bite out of my soap when I'm in the shower and have it stuck in my braces." But one of Pamela's most pressing concerns is not being able to drive:

> *I feel like I've missed out on a lot of things. I still feel that way because I have no transportation in the evening to do what I want to do like sing in my college's choir. I live nowhere close to our community college and the busses don't run at night. Everything else I'm fine but when it comes to transportation it's no fun.*[2]

Sean, whose epileptic seizures began when he was sixteen years old, also regretted not being able to drive. He says, "I'd been driving for close to a year, and a week after I got my license I was helping my mother drive cross-country. Driving was BIG, and after the seizure I had to be seizure free for a whole year before I could even THINK about driving again!"

LIFESTYLE CHANGES

Changes in daily living have a major impact on some people with epilepsy. As Lori Shively laments:

> *I have a dream to live a life without medication; I want to live a life of freedom; I want to live without the worry of not knowing when I'm going to have a seizure.*
> *You're afraid to go places by yourself most of the time. When you tell people you have seizures they kinda look at you strange and do everything possible to avoid you. What they don't realize is it hurts and we are just as afraid as they are!!*[3]

Other lifestyle changes may also be in order for a young person with epilepsy. Even if state laws permit drinking at age eighteen, for example, "You can't drink alcohol when you're taking an antiseizure medication like Dilantin," Sean notes. "Your liver is already working overtime to process the Dilantin, and alcohol just increases the workload. Add to that basic drug–alcohol interactions and you've got one recipe for trouble." Yet, he says,

I found several advantages to this forced sobriety. Although I didn't drink before I had epilepsy, the onset of seizures pretty much guaranteed that I would never start. Not being in conscious control of myself involuntarily has shown me that I don't want to get to that point voluntarily. I took advantage of this in an ironic way. I was able to go out with my friends who did drink. Even though I couldn't drive, I told the bartenders or servers that I was the designated driver and got my soft drinks for free. (In case you're wondering, the real driver would just nurse a single drink so it wouldn't affect him.) Of course, if you do get to drive again, you've gotten good practice in the art of identifying yourself as a designated driver.

Although the teenage years are a time for many to rebel and to assert their individuality, Sean warns a teenager with epilepsy: "DO NOT try to rebel by refusing to take your medication. Change your hairstyle, get something pierced, but take your prescribed medicine. Asserting your independence by choosing not to take your medication may, in the worst case, prevent you from becoming an adult, period. I tried to do that. All I got for my efforts to be independent was a seizure. I showed them: my timetable for being allowed to drive again got reset to zero. Yeah, I showed *them*!"

Another big change for Sean was to give up rowing on his school crew team. "My neurologist asked me to stop rowing until I went six months seizure free. That was tough. Rowing

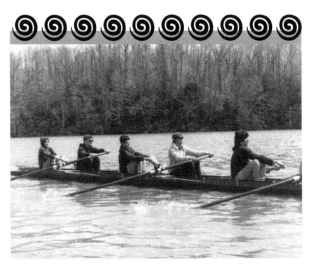

In this photo, Sean McGarrahan is practicing with his Citadel rowing team.

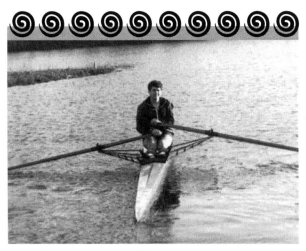

Sean McGarrahan is getting in shape for a team-rowing match.

had become a big part of my life. But if I couldn't row, then I was going to become a manager and learn all I could about the sport from the coaching side. I'm glad that I did that. I stayed connected with my teammates and was able to rejoin the team in the fall for my last season, after the requisite six months. That was the other reason for staying with the team. I had to keep my eye on a goal. Once I got back in the boat, my next milestone would be driving again."

Before that, however, Sean had to decide on a college. He wanted to go into the military like his father, but epilepsy prevented him from going to a service academy, which required an applicant to be seizure free for five years. "Fortunately," Sean says, "I found a college where I could get a military environment with the possibility of going into the military: The Citadel, The Military College of South Carolina. I was also fortunate that the school doctor was new and did not have a built-in prejudice against someone with epilepsy. He told me that the previous doctor would not have accepted me."

PARENTAL REACTIONS

When parents witness their child's seizure for the first time, the experience can be extremely frightening and shocking. One mother wrote about her thirteen-year-old daughter's first seizure followed by four others within a short time period: "I have never been as frightened as I was on that day. At first I thought she might die but as the seizures subsided, I realized that her life and ours would never be quite the same again."[4] Another mother wrote that her son's "first seizure scared me to pieces."[5]

Sean's father, John McGarrahan, a retired Army officer, described his reaction to his son's first seizure as "part of my memory like few other experiences." He and Sean were reading parts of the Sunday newspaper when, his father writes:

I heard a loud vocal sound, not a yell or shout, just an indistinct cry like a very noisy yawn coming from across the room. I looked over and saw Sean in a rigid position in the midst of a convulsion across the chair. He was shaking though not violently, and he did not seem to be aware of what he was doing. Soon he was lying on the floor, now moving around slightly erratically and gasping for air. As I first went over to him and talked to him, he really did not seem to be aware of me. I continued trying to talk with him, and soon he began to respond, but as if only half awake. That is, he seemed to know I was talking to him but really could not make sense of the words. Meanwhile, his mother had come into the room and I asked her to call 911 for an ambulance.

The five or fewer minutes of this experience seemed like hours on one hand yet like just seconds—all at the same time. My military experience kept my thoughts riveted on trying to "do something," even though I did not know exactly what. My heart, though, was saying "What is happening to my son?!" I had never seen someone experience a seizure before, so a sense of great concern jumped in quickly on top of being mystified. Fortunately, fear of him dying from this episode came and went quickly as he regained fuller awareness of where he was and began breathing more normally. So fear, then mystery, then concern, then questions, then different concerns all swirled around in me as we waited.[6]

Getting a diagnosis of epilepsy also creates alarm, fear, dread, and other negative reactions. Frequently parents say they have difficulty accepting the diagnosis. In some cases they don't really want to believe the doctors and are in denial at first. They may seek out support groups to help them deal with the reality.

In his book *Epilepsy and the Family*, Richard Lechtenberg, M.D., points out that parents of offspring who have seizures should have an accurate assessment of a young person's potential and should help him or her to "achieve that potential, both at school and at home." That, however, does not always happen. Some parents "impose excessive limits," such as not allowing their teenagers with epilepsy to engage in team sports. Other parents may feel guilty and believe they are "responsible for the affliction." Sometimes parents of epileptic offspring raise them to believe they are unable to accomplish much; as a result, by the time they are teenagers these young people have "inappropriate low aspirations and become very dependent on interpersonal relationships."[7]

On the other hand, as Sean put it:

I have been fortunate to have very loving and supportive parents. From the day that my parents witnessed my first seizure they have been supportive beyond anything I would have imagined at sixteen. No matter how they may have been feeling at the time, my parents never did anything that would increase my anxiety. Unless a desire of mine was specifically against doctor's orders or the law, my parents did not discourage me from my pursuits. From conversations I've had, I know my mother is very concerned about my bicycle riding, but although she tells me about the concern, she doesn't try to stop me.

FIRST AID

Not everyone who has a seizure needs first aid. Usually people who experience partial seizures and "blank out"

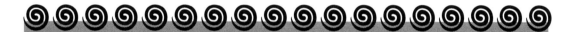

SEAN'S SEIZURE RECORD

To help in Sean's treatment, his father has kept a fairly detailed diary, or log, of each event. He has noted the length of the episode, the date and time, a description of the seizure, recovery time, some circumstances of the day, and his medication level. This record is the type that many doctors encourage epileptic patients to maintain. Because the log events date from 1985 to the present, only a few brief excerpts from it can be shown here:

19 Apr	1515	Citadel	In game room, playing pinball, alone. Awoke soon after, racketed by time points he recalled. Hit head hard, but no sign of concussion, per Dr. @ Chas. Navy. Phenobarbital level measured, barely therapeutic. Had not missed. Had been taking 500 mg Dilantin, 150 mg phenobarbital. Dr. @ ER directed change to 400 mg Dilantin, 180 mg phenobarbital.
25 Apr	1900	Charleston	At video store, Sz outside on sidewalk. Chipped/cracked tooth, bloody nose. Recovered fairly quickly. Called from Chas. Navy waiting for ER Dr. Had been taking 400 mg Dilantin, 180 mg phenobarbital.
10 May	1300–	Charleston	At Beach House. Had not missed. Had been taking 300 mg 1630 Dilantin, 180 mg phenobarbital. Was sleeping, wakened by phone, noted usual effects. Did not go to hosp.
31 Oct	0740	Apartment	Just after getting up. Up late night before at apartment working on paperwork and had not taken evening med.
7 Apr	? 1530	home	In computer room, while home sick. Fell forwards, hit face and chest on computer desk. Not feeling well for several days before.
14 Apr	0015	home	In bed, sleeping, after being up late. Recovery slow (17 minutes) before lucid. Had taken 300 mg Dilantin and 900 mg Neurontin about 2315 prior. Took another 200 mg dil and 200 mg neurontin at 0100. Upset stomach, no supper previous evening. Had taken normal doses previous morning and noontime. Took 300 mg Dilantin and 900 mg Neurontin at about 0800. At 0900, went to Springfield Kaiser-Perm. clinic to take Dilantin level. Level was 11.1 vice [10,20]. (15 Apr: Lipps decreased Neurontin to 1,800 mg/day and began Topamax, building to 200 mg/day over 4 weeks.)
2 May	0645	retreat	After shower shortly after getting up. Had not yet taken morning dose, but had taken 300 mg previous nite. On Monday, 4 May, went to Woodbridge Kaiser-Perm. Clinic and got Dilantin level taken. Level was 7.9 vice [10,20]. Dr. Lipps increased Dilantin to 650 mg/day.
7 May	1715	Work	At help desk office. Grazed face on computer keyboard. Had taken 200 mg Dilantin plus 900 mg Neurontin & 50 mg Topamax that morning. Had taken 200 mg Dilantin at 1230. Upset stomach and diar. after lunch. Recovered fairly quickly; he thought quicker. Went to Woodbridge Kaiser-Perm. Clinic and got Dilantin level taken. Level was ____ vice [10,20].
7 Oct	0830	home	In bathroom shortly after getting up. Fell, scraping back, left elbow. Recovered normally. Had just taken (0815) morning dose, but sure had taken 250 mg previous nite after 2300. Took another 200 mg after sz. Level taken?

only need emotional support and reassurance after they begin to respond to those around them. But what should be done when a person witnesses a tonic-clonic seizure? People having such seizures may fall; they may begin to jerk uncontrollably, foam at the mouth, and cry out. A first-time observer of a convulsion may become frightened and begin first aid that is based on false information. Many people believe a person will "swallow" his or her tongue during a seizure, so they put an object in a person's mouth. This is not only wrong, it's dangerous. The tongue cannot be swallowed, and the person having a seizure is likely to suffer a damaged mouth or broken teeth from the clenched object. In addition, a helper is likely to be bitten!

The kind of first aid that is helpful includes some simple dos and don'ts:

- Do place a pillow or other cushion under the person's head.
- Don't try to restrain a person; a seizure must end naturally.
- Do loosen tight neckwear.
- Don't leave a person alone; stay with him or her until the seizure ends.
- Do clear the area of sharp objects.
- Don't try to make the person drink anything.
- Do look for an epilepsy medical identification tag.

Sometimes helpers call 911 for an ambulance immediately, but experts say emergency service is not usually necessary. However, emergency assistance would be needed for a first generalized convulsion; if the seizure lasts more than five minutes; or if the person has repeated seizures without regaining consciousness, is pregnant, or has signs of injury.

SEIZURE-ALERT DOGS

In recent years, news stories, magazine articles, and Internet postings have described seizure-alert dogs, or companion dogs (and sometimes cats) that have the ability to sense and alert a person with epilepsy that she or he is about to have a seizure. Several minutes before a seizure happens, a dog may bark, paw, or circle around its owner. For example, Joel Davis wrote:

> *I have benefited from my dog Alex's ability in this area many times. Not only has he alerted me while I work at home, but even at times while we're out walking, if he detects an oncoming seizure, Alex will simply stop in his tracks and, despite the fact that I am considerably stronger than he is (Alex is a miniature Dachshund), he will not move another inch unless it is in the direction of our home.*[8]

Annie Cummins, who began having seizures after a car accident, learned for the first time that her dog, Adam, was able to alert her to a seizure. Adam "would be sleeping soundly then all of a sudden he would bark and bite at me. I thought he was nuts so I told him to go lay down and be quiet. The next thing I know he had his head on my lap and I was on the bed laying down," she wrote. In a later instance, she was driving her car with her dog asleep on the seat beside her. Then suddenly Adam awoke and Annie felt the dog looking at her. "I said, 'Good boy Adam, I understand.' With that I pulled over to the side of the road and shut the car off. He watched me for as long as I can remember. I remember him lying back down and that was it."

Because of her dog, Annie felt she could register for college in Colorado Springs, Colorado, and was accepted. "I would not have ventured out that far in the world if Adam hadn't given me the strength to," she wrote.[9]

The idea that a dog can detect the onset of a seizure before humans are able to do so is supported by anecdotal material, but few scientific studies have been able to show how an animal senses an oncoming seizure. In fact, the Epilepsy Foundation and the Epilepsy Institute caution that even though dogs may alert someone to the onset of a

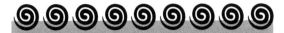

STORIES ON THE WEB

A web site that focuses on stories about seizure-alert and companion dogs can be accessed at http://members.tripod.com/~Ted_Bergeron/seizure-dog-index.html. Stories describe how dogs have protected people during seizures and have sometimes saved lives. Dogs may block falls and alert relatives, friends, or others that a person has had a seizure. One young woman who has daily seizures explains that she has a "Labrador retriever with topaz eyes, named Sugar." Sugar is a "specially trained service dog that alerts me anywhere from five minutes to an hour before a seizure occurs, and stays with me afterward until help arrives. [Sugar] has helped to give me new self-confidence and independence, because I never knew when or where I'd have a seizure."

seizure, there is no proof that an animal can be trained for this service.[10]

Researchers at the University of Florida's College of Veterinary Medicine have conducted surveys of people who have at least one seizure per month. Among them 69 percent had a dog and 11 percent of the owners "reported plausible alerting behavior by their dog." Thirty-three percent of owners said their dogs responded after their seizures began. In other words, the dogs remained beside their owner and provided comfort and some physical assistance. Such behavior can be trained. But, say the researchers, a dog's temperament and the "owner–dog bond" are significant in whether or not a dog will have seizure-alert abilities.[11]

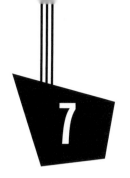

7 School and Job Issues

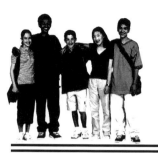

Along with changes in lifestyle and expectations, teenagers with epilepsy often must deal with uncertainty and anxiety. They wonder when the next seizure will occur. Will they be able to take part in school activities? Will they be able to get a driver's license? What about social events? A major concern is what others, especially friends and classmates, will think if they witness a seizure.

Eighteen-year-old Lisa Carney of Wichita, Kansas, says she has told her friends and others about her epilepsy since elementary school, when she often had seizures. She says when she mentioned seizures, the reaction she got was:

"What's that?" which was a little hard to explain being young, but I usually managed OK. Once I got to middle school I was tired of having to explain so I just didn't tell many people. I did tell my close friends, usually when they'd spend the night at my house, or I'd spend the night at their house and they'd see me taking pills. I just told them if I didn't take the pills I'd have seizures, some of them knew what that was, others needed more explanation.

Once I got to high school, it usually came up with some comment about my pills again. It had become so normal to just say "my pills" I forgot not everyone knew about that. So I'd have to explain why I took pills. Because my seizures are controlled, it wasn't an issue of having a seizure and then having to explain. I do have to explain the auras quite often though. That was interesting when I went to Spain with my classmates and out of a safety precaution I had to explain the whole thing to the entire group. J, my boyfriend, does know that if I forget my pills, I will probably have seizures. I have told

To help [young people] feel more confident about themselves and accept their epilepsy, the school can assist by providing epilepsy education programs for staff and students, including information on seizure recognition and first aid.

—National Information Center for Children and Youth with Disabilities

*him what happens and how to handle that. It used to
scare him or upset him, I'm not sure which one, but he
seems to be OK with it now.*[1]

Teenager Kristen Austin says that when her friends first
found out she had epilepsy

*they were kind of wary to be around me as if I would
break if they touched me. Some laughed at my seizures
because they were very abnormal. As an example of one,
I climbed onto my desk at school on day, lay down on it
and started "swimming" to the Agean Sea [sic] to visit
the penguins. So I was very frustrated when I found this
out because I was not completely conscious when this
was happening. I never knew what or when I would do
this. As the years went by I found out exactly who my
friends were, the ones who didn't tease me and stood up
for me are still my friends today.*[2]

SCHOOL PROBLEMS

When people have mistaken ideas about epilepsy, their reactions to seizures can sometimes be cruel and demeaning.
Some teenagers with epilepsy have reported instances of harassment, ridicule, and exclusion because they have had
seizures in public. One girl explained that her brother had a
seizure on the school bus. "When the other kids saw this they
started laughing, thinking he was joking around."[3] A mother
in central Florida said that when her son, David, was school
age, she had to defend him against neighborhood bullies who
feared and harassed David and threatened the family.

Adults, too, have misconceptions about epilepsy. It is not
unusual for school personnel to believe that a young person
having a seizure is "faking it" or "acting crazy" in an attempt to gain attention. Numerous young people with
epilepsy have been assigned to special education classes because teachers and other school personnel are irrationally
convinced that epilepsy is akin to mental retardation. As
Lisa noted, "When I was in elementary school, before the

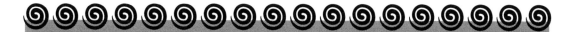

BILL OF RIGHTS

A web site sponsored by the Epilepsy Support for Youngsters and Teens contains a Bill of Rights for young people with epilepsy. Young people have contributed to the page, and any youth who has epilepsy can add an item to the Bill of Rights, which includes these statements:

We the young persons of this world who have epilepsy are entitled to the following rights:

I. No one should be teased or put down because of having epilepsy.

II. People with epilepsy should have the freedom to do what they want, without being turned away from certain things.

III. People with epilepsy should be able to talk about epilepsy without the fear of being ignored or put down for it.

IV. It is my right that my friends, acquaintances, teachers, coaches, etc., do not assume to understand my seizure disorder based upon their preconceived notions. Due to the many different seizures types and circumstances, I deserve the respect of being allowed to explain my seizure disorder or having my family or doctor doing so in my behalf.

V. No one can control when or where they are going to have a seizure and people should be sensitive and understanding to this, not get upset with them.

VI. Our parents must not be looked down by their employer for having to miss work in order to take care of us; without them we wouldn't have the strength to live for what we feel and have to live with for the rest of our lives.

VII. People with epilepsy deserve to be treated with dignity as do all human beings. Discrimination should not be tolerated in any case; the unborn, elderly, black, and white, we all have a common ground, and that is God.

VIII. People should be educated about epilepsy, since we are a great part of our society. The more we know about epilepsy, the less fear and shame we feel, the more we express our feelings about epilepsy, the more we are going to be accepted.

IX. We should be allowed to (age appropriate), as we are able to, make our own choices for what is right for our future.

X. You should not tell your parents they don't understand when they are the ones helping you.

XI. Parents shouldn't underestimate us and worry about us all the time. We are normal still, and deserve the freedom that kids [our] age normally have.[4]

seizures were controlled, the school personnel tried to put me in special-ed classes. But my dad fought that, because I was already working ahead of the class, and wasn't having problems."[5] Lisa, in fact, graduated with honors from the most challenging high school in her district.

Fear is also a common reaction for someone witnessing a seizure, especially for the first time. But as people learn more about epilepsy and seizures, they are not as likely to be frightened.

IGNORANCE
by
Lisa Carney
(a teenager with epilepsy)

They say "ignorance is bliss"
From what I can tell, they're wrong
Ignorance causes pain, fear, and even death
Not for the ignorant, though
The ignorant get a sense of power
From degrading those they don't understand
Maybe ignorance is fear
Fear of those not understood
And those not understood suffer
It's not their fault
They didn't ask to be different
Did you choose to be who you are?
No, it just happened
The ignorant don't understand that
And must make themselves stronger
Stronger and bigger by degrading others
Sometimes they don't realize it
Their ignorance has blinded them
To the hearts and pain of others
Maybe that's what they meant
When they said "ignorance is bliss"
(reprinted with permission)

DATING

Worries about dating and dating issues are common among teenagers, whether or not they have epilepsy. But concerns intensify when there's the possibility of having a seizure in public or while on a date. One teenager sought advice in a teen chat forum about how to deal with dating. She wrote: "I had a partial seizure when I was out at a friend's house recently. I was very embarrassed but everyone was really nice to me. It was not a grand mal, but I was out of it and didn't know what was going on." She explained that "a guy she really liked" asked her out, but she wasn't sure what to do.

Did you know? Like many teenagers, those with epilepsy may be involved in numerous activities and may be deprived of needed sleep. Sleep deprivation can trigger seizures in people with some forms of epilepsy, so it's important that teenagers with epilepsy get sufficient sleep on a regular basis.

Another teenager in the chat forum responded with an upbeat: "GO 4 IT. . . . Don't worry, guys understand."

Sixteen-year-old Kristin Austin says she has had no problems telling guys about her seizures. She says her current boyfriend "would always make sure I took my medication or made my doctors appointments, etc. He is very supportive and I love him very much for that."[6]

An eighteen-year-old advised telling "guys about it . . . tell them what the seizure looks like." She explained that her seizures were well controlled by medication, but she still tells dates "just in case" something happens. Her concluding words: "Epilepsy is a part of you, if they [guys] can't handle that, then they don't really care about you."[7]

That fact was made clear to Elizabeth Goodspeed. She explained in an *EpilepsyUSA* article that during high school she began having tonic-clonic and simple partial seizures and as a result "shut out the world. My guard was always up; my body language became inherently standoffish. Snubbing people was not my intent. In fact, what I needed was someone other than my parents to talk to, to cry to, and to understand what I was going through." Goodspeed noted that she especially feared dating because she "was scared.

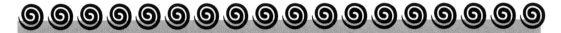

LEARNING DISABILITIES
WITH SEIZURE DISORDERS

The National Information Center for Children and Youth with Disabilities (NICHCY) points out that some students with epilepsy may have additional conditions such as learning disabilities along with the seizure disorders. These students are eligible for special education and related services under the Individuals with Disabilities Education Act (IDEA). In the organization's words:

> *Seizures may interfere with a student's ability to learn. If the student has the type of seizure characterized by a brief period of fixed staring, he or she may be missing parts of what the teacher is saying. It is important that the teacher observe and document these episodes and report them promptly to parents and to school nurses.*
>
> *Depending on the type of seizure or how often they occur, some [students] may need additional assistance to help them keep up with classmates. Assistance can include adaptations in classroom instruction, first-aid instruction on seizure management for the student's teachers, and counseling, all of which should be written in the IEP [Individualized Education Program].*
>
> *It is important that the teachers and school staff be informed about a [student's] condition, possible effects of medication, and what to do in case a seizure occurs at school. Most parents find that a friendly conversation with the teacher(s) at the beginning of the school year is the best way to handle the situation. . . . School personnel and the family should work together to monitor the effectiveness of medication as well as any side effects. . . . Students can benefit the most when both the family and school are working together.[8]*

I feared when and where I would have the next seizure, how severe it would be, who would see me, and mainly what they would think. I never know whether or not to tell the guy about my epilepsy, because I had myself convinced that he would leave right then." She also worried about whether anyone would ever marry her or want to have children with her.

For all her apprehensions, Goodspeed met a young man, Ed, who attended the same prep school as she, and the two began dating:

> *Early on in the relationship, I vividly recall deliberating whether or not to tell him that I have seizures. When I finally decided to, I was surprised at his response. He*

looked at me and simply stated, "I know that." Some of the guys in his dorm had had classes with me and had seen me have seizures. The fact that Ed was unfazed, that he had not been deterred, was initially shocking. The shock was short-lived, because as I came to know Ed better, I realized that the fact that I have epilepsy is not always a barrier.[9]

As Goodspeed and many others with epilepsy have learned, when a person feels okay talking about his or her seizures, others become comfortable. In general, people are usually interested in finding out what happens during a seizure, and friends, true friends, are understanding. Once it is clear that a person with epilepsy is not afraid of the disorder, others won't be either.

Did you know? Because of employers' false impressions about epilepsy, many workers with epilepsy are employed in jobs that are below their ability and educational levels, and their lifetime earnings are below the national average.

ON THE JOB

Teenagers (as well as adults) with epilepsy often have to face potential employers and co-workers who fear their seizures. Whether or not a person is hired or allowed to stay on the job depends on such factors as the type of work required, the type of epilepsy a person has, the frequency of seizures, the effects of medication, and a doctor's recommendation. For example, if a teenager has a pizza delivery job that requires driving and there's a chance of seizures, a job change will probably be necessary. But working in a fast-food restaurant would likely be possible, and office work shouldn't be a problem, assuming a teenager with epilepsy is not photosensitive and the computer screen doesn't trigger seizures.

Because of the misconceptions about epilepsy, teenagers with this disorder often wonder: Do I have to tell a job interviewer about my condition? If so, will that prevent me from being hired? Will co-workers freak out?

Lisa says that her experiences telling others about her epilepsy have varied with every job she's had. When she was on her first job, a co-worker fell and an ambulance was called. So Lisa took the opportunity to ask if anyone would know what to do if she had a seizure. No one had a clue, so "I did some explaining," Lisa said.

She now works two jobs, and before being hired for one position she mentioned her epilepsy during her interview. "Just in case anything happens," she told her employer. Lisa has also informed some of the managers on her other job, primarily because her doctor has been changing her medications and she wanted her co-workers to know there was a possibility she could have a seizure. In addition, her doctor is considering surgery for her, "and I wanted to talk about that," she said, which led to an interesting conversation with one of her supervisors.

Did you know? Former U.S. Congressman from California, Tony Coelho, who has epilepsy, was the primary author of the ADA. Coelho was honored for his efforts at a celebration in Washington, D.C., on ADA's tenth anniversary in 2000.

The supervisor "had a friend who had epilepsy and died in his sleep while having a seizure so it scares her more than others, but it's comforting to me to know that she understands." In conclusion, Lisa feels no obligation to tell her employers about her epilepsy, but she does so as a safety precaution, "just in case something were to happen—somebody should know."[10]

Some employers, however, may refuse to hire someone with epilepsy. One teenager, Jesse, tried to get a job at a grocery store that "hires teens to work every summer." But Jesse could not even get an application form. "They always tell me they are not hiring, but I've seen them the same day giving job applications to other teens. . . . Since I live in a small town, everyone knows I have epilepsy and have to use a wheelchair sometimes to get around (if I have a seizure that is bad, I can't walk well afterward)," Jesse reported.[11]

In this instance, the employer may have been violating a federal law: the Americans with Disabilities Act (ADA).

The Act protects people with epilepsy and requires employers to consider hiring anyone who is qualified and able to perform the essential job functions. The employer must make reasonable accommodations so that there is equal opportunity in the application process, in performing essential functions of the position, and in enjoying equal benefits and privileges of employment that are enjoyed by employees without disabilities. The reasons for and purposes of the Act are detailed in the appendix.

Certainly employers have legitimate concerns about whether a person with epilepsy will be injured because of seizures in the workplace and whether absenteeism, liability risks, and insurance rates will increase. Nevertheless, employers, like others in the general public, frequently are uneducated about epilepsy. In addition, teenagers looking for their first jobs may be unfamiliar with the protections spelled out in the ADA. Or they may be shy, lack confidence in their own abilities, or if they can't drive, believe they will be unable to find dependable transportation to the job.

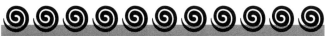

JOB COUNSELING

Some young people with epilepsy seek help from job counselors such as those at various Epilepsy Foundation offices in the United States and similar facilities in Canada. Tim Nourse, an employment consultant at Epilepsy Toronto (Canada), points out a common problem for clients looking for work: fear of seizures on the job. Nourse tells the young people he counsels to "inform those around you at work, church, school, sports team, family and friends, that this is what the seizure looks like and this is the type of support I need or, perhaps more importantly, don't need. Wear medical identification. This may reduce the fear of seizures because the individual will know that they will occur but they can be managed."

Yet, Nourse says if a person has a tonic-clonic seizure and falls, there can be significant head trauma, "bones can be fractured and dislocated, soft tissue can be damaged often resulting in disfiguring scars (try explaining the black eye or stitched cheek to co-workers after a long weekend)."

Nourse says that his agency sees "too many people in vocational crisis. They have a seizure on the job and are about to lose the job or have lost it already." The clients Nourse and others in the agency see may or may not have disclosed their epilepsy to the employer prior to the seizure. Sometimes disclosure "doesn't seem to matter," Nourse says. To assist in such instances, Nourse or others in the agency may approach the employer on the client's behalf and "and facilitate dialog or if it appears that a stronger approach is needed," the agency may help a client file a complaint with a human rights authority.[12]

In 2000, the U.S. Department of Labor provided a grant of $350,000 for the Epilepsy Foundation of America to launch a three-year experiment, called JobTech. The program is under way at Epilepsy Foundation affiliates in

Camden, New Jersey; Mobile, Alabama; Rockford, Illinois; and Kansas City, Missouri. Through the program teenagers and adults with epilepsy can learn computer skills and such techniques as how to write effective resumes, search for jobs, and develop interview skills.

JobTech programs hope to prepare participants for a variety of jobs, including computer programming, systems analysis, sales and customer service, process control operations, and other positions that call for computer skills. The programs will help place people in positions such as retail clerk, administrative assistant, web page specialist, customer service representative, computer technician, electronic data processing, bank teller, data entry clerk, and billing clerk.

Did you know? Studies show that workers with epilepsy and those without the disorder don't differ in accident and absenteeism rates and job performance. If there are safety concerns on the job, some simple accommodations may enable the person with epilepsy to perform the work effectively and safely.

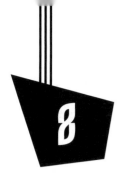

8

Sports and Recreation

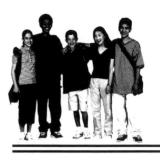

Most people with controlled seizures can take part in a variety of sports and recreational activities. Taylor, a teenager writing for an epilepsy web site, noted: "I've had epilepsy all my life, but I accept what I have, and live with it. I am in many activities. . . . I play in our high school band, JV Baseball, I am the catcher, and I am in many clubs."[1]

Team and individual sports play an important role in the lives of many young people with epilepsy. Even a person who has seizures once a week may take part in sports and recreation, because she or he still has 313 seizure-free days in the year, notes the American College of Physicians. "It is thus important that a person does not let the epilepsy take over and control his or her life. Overprotection, excessive restrictions, and underachievement are far too common secondary handicaps of epilepsy, and they can be avoided."[2]

Certainly some risks also have to be avoided. People with epilepsy are advised not to take part in such sports as motor racing, skydiving, hang gliding, scuba diving, recreational flying, and other activities that require concentration at all times. Mountain climbing can pose hazards as well. "It's not only the risk of falling if you should have a seizure, the reduced oxygen and atmospheric changes at the kind of elevations encountered in some kinds of mountain climbing may increase seizure risk, too," cautions the Epilepsy Foundation.

Sports such as bicycling, swimming, boating, and horseback riding are relatively safe for a person who has seizures, but precautions should be taken, such as wearing a helmet while bicycling or horseback riding, alerting a lifeguard before swimming, and boating only with another person along.

Leading an active life is good medicine for most people with epilepsy. . . . The Epilepsy Foundation encourages people with epilepsy to engage in sports and recreation activities as part of a positive approach to an active life.

—Epilepsy Foundation

63

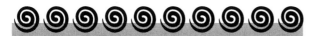

SUMMER CAMPS

During the summer, camps offering a variety of recreational and sports activities for young people with epilepsy are conducted in various parts of the United States. While some of the camps are geared for preteens, others are for teenagers and young adults. For example, Camp Ozawizeniba (Oz, for short) in Minnesota is a week-long overnight camp for young people with epilepsy ages eight to seventeen. Camp Blackhawk is a six-day residential camp held at Timber Pointe Camp near Hudson, Illinois, for those ages eight to sixteen who have epilepsy. In New Jersey, Camp Nova is a epilepsy and developmental disability camp for ages eight to twenty-five.

Some typical activities at epilepsy camps include horseback riding, boating, swimming, fishing, cookouts, evening campfires with singing, skits, organized games, and discussion groups, which are of particular interest to teenagers. Usually registered nurses, a neurologist, and other medical personnel are on staff.

Camps for young people with epilepsy are sponsored by affiliates of the Epilepsy Foundation of America in states ranging from New York to Washington, Florida to Wisconsin. *Epilepsy-USA* publishes an annual list of various camps along with their phone numbers and costs.

A CHAMPION SWIMMER

It's not unusual when a person with epilepsy takes up swimming as a sport. But it is unusual when a person with epilepsy also is paralyzed from the chest down and despite the physical handicap becomes a competitive swimmer, winning numerous medals. Such a person is Margaret McEleny of Greenock, Scotland.

During the 1970s, McEleny was injured while playing netball (a game similar to basketball) in high school. A metal bar supporting a net toppled and struck McEleny on the head; the injury led to seizures. Several years later, she had a seizure on an escalator and as a result of the accident suffered status epilepticus and went into a coma. After a month, she came out of the coma, but was paralyzed from the neck down.

There was a long period of therapy and a battle with depression, but McEleny recovered movement in her arms and was able to get around in a wheelchair. She was determined to get on with her life, "to make the best of what I had left," she told staff at *EpilepsyUSA*.

Swimming became part of McEleny's physical rehabilitation and she soon began to train with a coach for competition. Since 1992, she has competed in Paralympic Games and European and World Swimming Championships, winning gold, silver, and bronze medals and breaking world records for the breast stroke. Even though she has a tonic-clonic seizure about once a week, she has been able to safely continue training and competing. "When

I'm training, I always have someone there to watch. If they see anything different in my stroke, they call for a lifeguard. Having someone there with me is how I carry on with this sport," she told a reporter.[3]

BIKING FOR EPILEPSY

Many people who have epilepsy and are restricted from driving or operating other vehicles use a bicycle as a means of transportation. But one man, John O'Grady, a former pilot for United Parcel Service and recreational and professional balloonist, has used his bicycle for another purpose: He has biked thousands of miles to raise public awareness about epilepsy. Why? Because O'Grady had a tonic-clonic seizure in April 2000, and since then his whole life has changed.

O'Grady of Dayton, Ohio, grew up always wanting to fly—his father was a pilot and his mother a flight attendant. His flying career began with Airborne Express, and later he "moved to United Parcel Service to fly as an international captain on the B757/767," he writes. "I loved my career. I have enjoyed travels that took me to the farthest corners of the world, spectacular views from the cockpit, and memories to last a lifetime. I couldn't imagine doing anything else, and planned to continue flying until I retired." He also flew hot air balloons, taking people on balloon rides and competing in balloon competitions across the United States. "I learned how to fly with precision; flying to a target or a big X on the ground using only the

On its Internet web site, the Epilepsy Foundation posts these ideas about recreation safety for people with epilepsy:

Safer Recreation

- When exercising, take frequent breaks, stay cool, and save your greatest exertion for the coolest part of the day.
- Exercise on soft surfaces if you can—grass, mats, wood chips.
- Review the risks carefully before taking up sports which could put you in danger if you were suddenly unaware of what you were doing.
- Wearing a life vest is a good idea when you are on or close to water.
- Swimming can be safe and fun for everyone, but if you have seizures, avoid swimming alone.
- Tell lifeguards and friends you swim with what kind of seizures you have, how to recognize them, and what to do if you have one. Make sure they swim well enough to help if you need it.
- Wear head protection when playing contact sports or when there is an added risk of falling or head injuries.
- If you ski or hike, go with a buddy; you may need someone to get help if you have a seizure in remote areas.
- Consider use of a safety strap and hook when riding the ski lift.[4]

wind to navigate there. I qualified in the top 100 USA pilots allowing me to fly four times in the National Championships," O'Grady writes.[5]

When O'Grady had his seizure he had just completed an international flight and was on his way home. He stopped for breakfast and the next thing he knew he was waking up in a hospital near Cincinnati. He was diagnosed with epilepsy. As he reported:

> *I had no idea what Epilepsy was, but as a pilot . . . I knew that if I had a seizure, I would not be able to fly airplanes or hot air balloons. In what seemed like the blink of an eye, I lost my FAA medical certificate, 23-year career of flying the world, my hot air balloon business of 17 years, and cannot even drive a car. . . . I began riding my bike everywhere and have turned my only mode of transportation into my passion. I have traveled to Albuquerque [New Mexico] for many years in the past to compete in the biggest balloon rally in the world. Since I couldn't fly a balloon . . . I decided [in 2000] to ride my bicycle from Dayton, Ohio, to Albuquerque. I wanted to put my cycling to good use and raise money in the process for three nonprofit organizations: Pilots for Kids, Jr. Balloonist, and The Epilepsy Foundation of Western Ohio. This was not only a personal challenge but also gave me a chance to raise awareness of epilepsy along the way. The ride was a success![6]*

On September 23, 2001, O'Grady began another bicycle trip from Dayton, Ohio, to Las Vegas, Nevada, arriving on October 24, 2001, at the MGM Grand Hotel in Las Vegas for a weekend Epilepsy Foundation National Conference. He had biked more than 2,400 miles through Ohio, Indiana, Kentucky, Tennessee, Alabama, Mississippi, Arkansas, Texas, New Mexico, Arizona, and Nevada. (Photos and details about his trip are available on a Web site: <http://johnscharityride.joesacher.com>.)

During his bike ride, O'Grady made numerous stops to visit schools and discuss epilepsy with students. On a stop in Tennessee, O'Grady met with nineteen-year-old Ben Marlow, who had earned his private pilot's license, but just months afterward was diagnosed with epilepsy. Marlow had written to O'Grady explaining how his dream to be a pilot was shattered. As Marlow put it:

I dreamed of flying night and day until I was a senior in high school. . . . So the day after I graduated from high school, I took a flying lesson in Knoxville, Tennessee. From the moment we took off, I was hooked. I finally could get my dad off my back about what I wanted to do with my life . . . I wanted to be a professional airplane pilot. After 5 months of flying just about every day, I received a Private Pilot License on October 22, 2000. It was the happiest day of my life. I was seriously on my way to doing what I love for a career! I was a pilot!

But that all came crashing down in March of 2001, when I was getting ready to come back to school [college] from a weekend at home. I was doing my laundry, and the next thing I knew, I was being loaded onto an ambulance. After 2 days of testing at St. Mary's Medical Center in Knoxville, the EEG results were back and they were not good. After 3 EEG's and 2 abnormal readings, I was diagnosed with epilepsy and told I had a petit mal or complex partial seizure. I felt so helpless, because this was something I couldn't fight off. As with many people I went through the "denial" stage. I had a very difficult time with the "why me?" stage. It was all over. The flying, the scuba diving, just about all I do. That was all until I heard about the story of John O'Grady [in] EpilepsyUSA, a magazine that my dad brought back from a support group meeting that I did not attend because I was going through the denial and didn't believe I had epilepsy. That [story] totally changed my outlook, as there was someone else in the same situation as me, whereas before, I felt alone.

Marlow was able to get in touch with O'Grady by e-mail and asked his advice. O'Grady responded with words that Marlow says he "will never forget," telling him, "Flying is what we did, not who we are." "Mr. O'Grady has inspired me to have a more positive outlook at the situation than I did before."[7]

Ben Marlow has followed O'Grady's example and is going on with his life. Not only is he planning a different career but he is also speaking out about epilepsy in order to raise awareness about the disorder.

THE JADE FOUNDATION

Sports and recreation—from basketball to horseback riding to fishing—are part of Jade Ventura's life. Jade, who has epilepsy, is the teenage daughter of Governor Jesse Ventura and First Lady Terry Ventura of Minnesota, who founded the Jade Foundation to benefit young people with disabilities in their state.

Jade began having seizures not long after she was born in 1983. Although her seizures subsided, they began again when she was still an infant. The seizures caused permanent brain damage. But over the years, Jade has received "all kinds of therapy," and is a successful student and athlete in suburban Minneapolis–St. Paul. Her mother proudly relates on a web site for the foundation:

> She can drive wave-runners (personal watercraft) and she is just learning to handle our John Deere tractor at the ranch. Soon she will start her driver's permit training. She plays the piano and the flute, and sings in the school choir. She played basketball on school teams almost every year (including two championship basketball teams).

Jade also loves horses and rides for pleasure and in shows. Terry Ventura notes that Jade has a can-do spirit and "loves to learn and experience new things." Special education programs in Minnesota have been a great help in Jade's progress. But, Terry Ventura adds, Jade "is also the product of intense parental involvement, lots of love from her big brother, support of her friends, and care and attention from her extended family."[8]

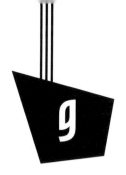

9 The Female Factor

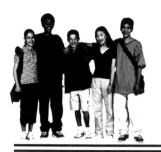

Girls and women with epilepsy sometimes face more complex health care issues than do males with seizure disorders. Many teenage girls wonder how drugs will affect them as women. For example, girls with epilepsy may experience more frequent seizures around the time of their menstrual periods. Antiseizure medications may also interfere with hormone regulation and can reduce the effectiveness of birth control pills.

Females with epilepsy are more prone to reproductive problems than are those who do not have seizure disorders. They may be at risk for cysts on the ovaries, a condition known as polycystic ovaries (PCO), which may affect fertility—whether someone is able to become pregnant.

> **Did you know? About one million American teenage girls and women live with epilepsy.**

TEENAGE CHANGES

Hormonal changes, particularly during the teenage years, can have a direct effect on someone with epilepsy. Hormones are chemical substances in the body secreted from endocrine glands. They control or influence such processes as muscle growth, heart rate, behavior, the reproductive system, and the menstrual cycle. During puberty, hormones stimulate body changes and may affect certain types of seizures. Some seizures that begin in childhood may disappear at puberty, while other types may begin at this time of hormonal changes.

Many teenage girls as well as women with epilepsy "receive their treatment from primary care and community physicians who may not be aware of recent information showing that infertility and menstrual disturbances may be associated with some antiepileptic drugs."

—Martha Morrell, Professor of Neurology at Columbia University College of Physicians & Surgeons and Director of the Columbia Comprehensive Epilepsy Center of New York–Presbyterian Hospital

The connection between seizures and hormones is not yet well understood. But according to the Epilepsy Foundation,

> *The female hormones, estrogen and progesterone, act on certain brain cells, particularly those in the temporal lobe, a part of the brain where partial seizures often begin. Estrogen excites these brain cells and can make seizures more likely to happen. In contrast, progesterone can inhibit or prevent seizures in some [cases]. The temporal lobes are closely connected to, and communicate with, areas of the brain that regulate hormones (hypothalamus and pituitary gland). Seizures in these areas may affect normal production of hormones.*[1]

CATAMENIAL EPILEPSY

Catamenial epilepsy refers to seizures that are more frequent or severe during the menstrual cycle. Patterns of seizure frequency and severity are related to the level of certain reproductive hormones in the blood, according to the Weill Cornell Department of Neurology and Neuroscience at Cornell University. The department is conducting a study sponsored by the National Institutes of Health (NIH) to evaluate the effect of treating seizures that are related to menstruation with progesterone. The hormone progesterone has been shown to have an anti-seizure effect and may be helpful for some epileptic females.

Did you know? People with epilepsy have lower birth rates than those without the disorder, which is due to such factors as lack of sexual drive, reduced fertility, and social pressures *not* to have children.

Teenage and adult women are treated at the Comprehensive Epilepsy Center of New York Hospital–Cornell Medical Center. A neuroendocrinologist, a specialist who deals with the interrelationships between hormones and the brain, guides the treatment of those with catamenial epilepsy.

PREGNANCY CONCERNS

It's not unusual for teenage girls with epilepsy to worry about their future as mothers. Should they have children? Even if they don't have epilepsy, maybe a partner does. Would that mean that their child might inherit a seizure disorder? Or teenagers with epilepsy might be concerned that if they become parents, they will have seizures and endanger their children while caring for them.

Some teenagers with epilepsy believe they will never be able to have children, or they have been advised by relatives, friends, or even their doctors not to get pregnant because their children may suffer birth defects. They may be alarmed by reports from women who make comments like this: "I would like to have a child one day but the thought of coming off my medication terrifies me as does the thought of the side effects the medication could have on a child."[2]

On the other hand, teenagers may be reassured by messages such as one posted on an Internet forum by a woman who wrote that she and her husband consulted neurologists before she got pregnant. "The first neurologist I spoke with had me convinced that we should never have children since my seizure medication is considered highly teratogenic [causes birth defects]. . . . I did not go off medication. We spoke with some terrific neurologists who were willing to take time with us and show us actual research statistics concerning my meds, etc. With their help and the help of my OB [obstetrician], we decided to have our two wonderful children."[3]

The Epilepsy Foundation in its *Report to the Nation* states that "well managed pregnancies can have excellent outcomes."[4] An important factor in childbearing is not the epilepsy itself, but the medication taken to control seizures.

Antiseizure medication should be taken during pregnancy, but some drugs can increase the risk of such birth defects as cleft lip or palate. The risk of having a baby with certain kinds of birth defects is 4 to 6 percent among pregnant females with epilepsy compared with a rate of 2 to 3 percent of those in the general population.

Whether or not they are pregnant, all female patients of childbearing age should take folic acid supplements, doctors advise; the supplements reduce the risk of spina bifida and other neural tube defects (NTDs), and folic acid works best if patients are on it at the time of conception.

Because of the high rate of teenage pregnancies in the United States and the fact that most are unintended, folic acid supplements are an important part of any regimen for teenage girls, especially those with epilepsy.

More than a decade ago, the U.S. Centers for Disease Control and Prevention (CDC) and the U.S. Public Health Service began an educational campaign to encourage all teenagers of reproductive age and women to age forty-five to take folic acid in vitamin supplements and to eat foods fortified with folic acid. In mid-2001, the CDC reported a 19 percent decrease in neural tube defects because of folic acid fortification in the U.S. food supply.[5]

Did you know? The United States has the highest rate of teenage pregnancies of any industrialized nation. Although the teenage birth rates began to fall in the 1990s, each year about one million teenage girls between ages fifteen and nineteen in the United States become pregnant and about half that number become mothers.

BEFORE AND DURING PREGNANCY

All adolescents who become pregnant should get proper medical care early in their pregnancies. And any female of childbearing age with epilepsy should consult her obstetrician or family physician before deciding to become pregnant, experts say. With prenatal counseling, a doctor can explain possible health risks and change antiseizure medications if necessary. In addition, vitamin supplements, particularly folic acid, can be started before conception, reducing risks of birth defects.

Pregnancy may bring changes in seizures. About 30 percent of epileptic females experience an increase in seizures while pregnant; 20 percent have fewer seizures. There are no changes in seizure patterns for the remaining 50 percent of pregnant females with epilepsy.[7]

It is not clear why a pregnancy can sometimes increase seizures. Some experts theorize that antiseizure medication may not be as effective because of increased blood volume during pregnancy, which can decrease the levels of anticonvulsants in the blood. Elevated estrogen levels may play a role, and not getting enough sleep may also be a factor in increased seizures. Doctors advise anyone with epilepsy (pregnant or not) to get plenty of sleep and to have their blood levels of seizure medication monitored. Dosages of medications can be adjusted if necessary.

During the final month of pregnancy, vitamin K supplements may be in order. Antiseizure medications decrease the amount of vitamin K in the body, and the vitamin is

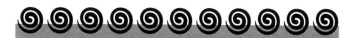

NTDS, RISK PREVENTION, AND FOLIC ACID

About four to six weeks after conception, the neural tube forms in the embryo (developing baby) and then closes. The neural tube later becomes the baby's spinal cord, spine, brain, and skull. A neural tube defect (NTD) occurs when the neural tube fails to close properly, leaving the developing brain or spinal cord exposed to the amniotic fluid. The two most common neural tube defects are anencephaly and spina bifida.

Anencephaly is a fatal condition in which the upper end of the neural tube fails to close, and the brain either never completely develops or is totally absent. Pregnancies affected by anencephaly often result in miscarriages.

Spina bifida occurs when the lower end of the neural tube fails to close. Thus, the spinal cord and back bones do not develop properly. Sometimes, a sac of fluid protrudes through an opening in the back, and a portion of the spinal cord is often contained in this sac. Paralysis of the infant's legs, loss of bowel and bladder control, water on the brain (hydrocephalus), and learning disabilities are among the disabilities associated with spina bifida.

To prevent NTDs, the U.S. Centers for Disease Control, the Food and Drug Administration, and numerous other health organizations recommend that all females of childbearing age (not just those with epilepsy) consume 400 micrograms (0.4 milligrams) of folic acid every day. Folic acid is a B vitamin and is found in folic acid pills and multivitamin tablets. It is also in fortified breakfast cereals such as Total, Product 19, Cheerios Plus, and Smart Start, and in enriched grain products such as pasta and rice. Foods containing folate include fruits and orange juice from concentrate; green, leafy vegetables; and dried beans and legumes. Folic acid in a vitamin supplement, when taken one month before conception and throughout the first trimester, has been proven to reduce the risk for an NTD-affected pregnancy by 50 to 70 percent.[6]

needed to help prevent bleeding problems in infants. New-borns may also be given vitamin K to ensure proper blood clotting.

How do epilepsy medications affect a baby? "Babies sometimes have symptoms of withdrawal from the mother's seizure medications after they are born, but these problems wear off in a few weeks or months and usually do not cause serious or long-term effects," states the NINDS. Only small amounts of antiseizure drugs are secreted in breast milk, so there is seldom any harm done if a mother decides to breast feed her baby.[8]

Research on how antiseizure medications affect the off-spring of epileptic females is under way at the Genetics and Teratology Unit of the Massachusetts General Hospital. The hospital has established a national registry for teenage and adult women who take antiseizure medication while preg-nant. Anyone enrolled in the program receives "educational materials on pre-conception planning and perinatal care and are asked to provide [confidential] information about the health of their children."[9] This will help researchers learn how certain drugs affect a fetus.

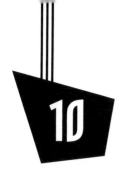

Finding a Cure

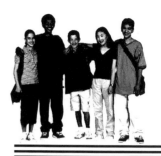

In 2000 the National Institute of Neurological Disorders and Stroke of the National Institutes of Health sponsored a conference called "Curing Epilepsy: Focus on the Future." The conference brought together leading scientists to discuss how epilepsy may be prevented and cured in the future.

Did you know? An old superstition says that the purple flower in the center of the wild carrot, also known as Queen Anne's lace, would help cure epilepsy.

When it comes to the treatment of epilepsy, the science fiction of today is the reality of tomorrow.

—Timothy A. Pedley, M.D., Columbia-Presbyterian Medical Center

At the present time, brain surgery is the only way that people with some types of epilepsy can become seizure free. But only a few thousand of the 2.5 million Americans with epilepsy are candidates for surgery. Thus, others must depend on drug therapy or wait for researchers to develop new treatments. Support for research, however, depends on public awareness of what epilepsy is and how it affects those with the disorder.

AWARENESS PROGRAMS

Various U.S. organizations have conducted programs in recent years to inform the public about epilepsy and ongoing research. Citizens United for Research in Epilepsy (CURE), for example, is a grassroots organization that works to stimulate research on epilepsy and publicize the need for a cure. The National Institute of Neurological Disorders and Stroke (NINDS) supports research on disorders of the brain and nervous system and sponsors a public information program about research related to seizures and epilepsy.

The main epilepsy organization in the United States is the Epilepsy Foundation. With its affiliates in more than 100 communities across the nation, the Foundation conducts numerous campaigns to raise awareness about epilepsy. One example is the Teen Awareness Campaign, funded by the U.S. Centers for Disease Control and Prevention. The Foundation hopes to reach "the general teen population . . . at the very crucial time they are beginning to form important attitudes and beliefs, as well as health habits and behaviors."

As part of the Teen Awareness Campaign, Epilepsy Month in November 2001 was dedicated to teenagers. The theme "Entitled to Respect" featured information about epilepsy and how teenagers deal with the disorder. Stories about teens with epilepsy appeared in varied media and special messages featured the concept of respect for teens with epilepsy.

Did you know? Epilepsy Foundation affiliates across the United States surveyed more than 19,400 teenagers and found that just over half of the teens (52 percent) who responded had ever heard of or read about epilepsy. The majority did not know whether epilepsy was contagious.

A POSSIBLE BRAIN "SWITCH"

Over the past decade, research has been under way that might one day make surgical removal of parts of the brain unnecessary. Researchers in several fields—neuroscience, mathematics, and biophysics—are conducting experiments to learn whether "nonlinear dynamics" can help in developing a switch or electrical device that could avert epileptic seizures.

Nonlinear dynamics is a theoretical branch of mathematics that is based on the fact that diverse systems ranging from ocean wave patterns to interplanetary movements exhibit similar, sometimes even universal behavior patterns. Researchers are applying the theory to help them understand the interconnected system of neurons in the brain.

The research differs from traditional neuroscience studies; rather than study the details of, for example, groups of neurons in the brain, the focus is on identifying large-scale patterns of interacting neurons. This could lead to controlling the bursts of electrical activity that occur in the brain during a seizure.

"The dynamic that generates the burst [of electricity] is much simpler than what all of the individual actors [parts of the brain] are doing," according to Dr. Bruce J. Gluckman, who leads the study at George Mason University in Virginia.[1] The research is expected to lead to a technique whereby a device with electrodes could be implanted in the brain to detect the onset of a seizure and then apply electrical charges that could redistribute electrical activity in neurons and ward off an electrical storm.

GENE RESEARCH

Gene research that is under way through the Human Genome Project could contribute to epilepsy research, scientists say. Some of the tools in gene research are microarrays, or "gene chips," which provide information on many different genes.

"Identifying the genes involved in epilepsy will contribute to an understanding of the neurochemical events involved in the development of the disorder and, in turn, to new opportunities for pharmacological [drug] intervention," according to a report in the *Journal of the American Medical Association*. Gene identification could help determine which drugs are most likely to be successful in treating people with epilepsy rather than using the trial-and-error procedure that is now usually required. "The hope is that new anticonvulsant compounds can be developed that will minimize adverse effects of the current drugs, which occur because the drugs affect the entire brain. More narrowly targeted agents, or devices that can deliver drugs directly to the areas involved, could minimize these effects."[2]

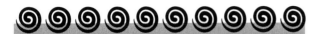

PLAYING VIDEO GAMES FOR SCIENCE

Video games and a science investigation may not seem like a likely combination. But in 1999 teenagers with severe epilepsy who could not be adequately treated with medication took part in a study conducted by researchers at Brandeis University and Children's Hospital in Massachusetts. The study examined the electrical activity in the teenagers' brains as they maneuvered through the game's virtual mazes. The researchers focused on slow, rhythmic waves of electrical activity known as theta oscillations.

The game was created by a fifteen-year-old high school student specifically for this research. In a virtual environment, such as found in popular video games, players were led through the mazes and then had to find their own way through a sometimes baffling set of twists and turns. To be successful, players had to remember where they'd been and how they got there.

With careful attention to the teenagers' safety, wires were attached directly on the surface of the teenagers' brains, and then connected to a monitor. The researchers could watch the electrical signals while the teens worked their way through the mazes. They found that various parts of the brain produced episodes of theta oscillations that were most pronounced when the teenagers were wending their way through extremely difficult mazes.

The study is just one of many that scientists have conducted in order to understand why the brain's rhythmic activity sometimes spins out of control. As researchers continue to study the findings, they may eventually discover how memory works and ultimately help develop a cure for epilepsy.[3]

CLINICAL TRIALS

As with other medical studies, clinical trials are an essential part of epilepsy research. Through clinical trials, new therapies can be tested and compared with standard treatments, helping researchers to develop better methods to more effectively treat individuals. For example, numerous research studies involving teenagers and adults newly diagnosed with seizures are being conducted across the nation in such states as Alabama, Connecticut, California, Georgia, Illinois, Massachusetts, New York, Ohio, and Texas. The types of trials currently recruiting patients can be found on web sites sponsored by hospitals, pharmaceutical companies, neurological centers, ClinicalTrials.gov sponsored by the NINDS, and CenterWatch (www.centerwatch.com).

Anyone who considers taking part in a clinical trial should understand what the study is about and what will be expected of a participant. In the first place, a person has to volunteer for a clinical trial and meet certain criteria. For example, only female volunteers with epilepsy take part in trials being conducted by the Neuroendocrine Unit at Beth Israel Deaconess Center in Boston, Massachusetts. The purpose of one study is to determine if there are differences in the types of seizures experienced by those who take progesterone and those who do not take the hormone. Another trial study is investigating how the brain changes during the menstrual cycle.

An individual who participates in a clinical trial must be given informed consent forms. The informed consent process means that a person receives written information that describes the purpose of the study; risks and benefits of being in the study; and what will happen during the study.

One clinical trial sponsored by NINDS is recruiting volunteers in order to examine the safety and effectiveness of infusing a chemical called muscimol into the brain to control seizures in patients with intractable epilepsy (frequent seizures that persist despite therapy). Muscimol, which is similar to a naturally occurring brain chemical called GABA, has been shown to reduce seizures in rats. After the infusion study, patients will undergo a standard surgical procedure for controlling seizures. Patients must be at least eighteen years of age with intractable epilepsy to be eligible for this study. Any candidate will be screened through such procedures as physical and neurologic examinations, a chest X-ray, electrocardiogram, blood and urine tests, electroencephalographic (EEG) monitoring, and magnetic resonance imaging (MRI) of the head.

The possible risks of being involved in a clinical trial depend on the study. Perhaps there will be adverse side effects from taking a medication being tested, or a patient might have to pay for some treatments.

On the other hand, the benefits of taking part in a clinical trial include getting free health examinations, learning more about one's own health, taking an active role in health care, and being closely monitored for health problems. Finally, a person with epilepsy who participates in a clinical trial helps researchers answer questions that may mean better health for epileptic patients in the future.

The prospects for advances in epilepsy research have never been better, say the experts, and they call on not only scientists but also the drug industry and the public to support research efforts. Such efforts encourage people with epilepsy and their relatives and friends to maintain hope that there will soon be a medical breakthrough for a cure.

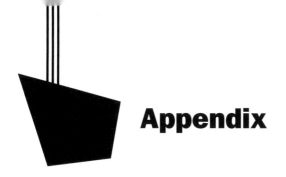

Appendix

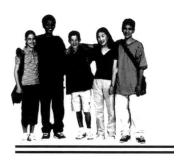

Epilepsy is considered a disability under the Americans with Disabilities Act (ADA). The Act requires employers to consider hiring anyone who is qualified and able to perform the essential job functions. The employer must make reasonable accommodations so that there is equal opportunity in the application process, in performing essential functions of the position, and in enjoying equal benefits and privileges of employment that are enjoyed by employees without disabilities.

The reasons (findings) for the law and its purposes are contained in Section 2 of the Act.

AMERICANS WITH DISABILITIES ACT OF 1990
SEC. 2. FINDINGS AND PURPOSES.

(a) Findings.—The Congress finds that—

(1) some 43,000,000 Americans have one or more physical or mental disabilities, and this number is increasing as the population as a whole is growing older;

(2) historically, society has tended to isolate and segregate individuals with disabilities, and, despite some improvements, such forms of discrimination against individuals with disabilities continue to be a serious and pervasive social problem;

(3) discrimination against individuals with disabilities persists in such critical areas as employment, housing, public accommodations, education, transportation, communication, recreation, institutionalization, health services, voting, and access to public services;

(4) unlike individuals who have experienced discrimination on the basis of race, color, sex, national origin, religion, or age, individuals who have experienced discrimination on the basis of disability have often had no legal recourse to redress such discrimination;

(5) individuals with disabilities continually encounter various forms of discrimination, including outright intentional exclusion, the discriminatory effects of architectural, transportation, and communication barriers, overprotective rules and policies, failure to make modifications to existing facilities and practices, exclusionary qualification standards and criteria, segregation, and relegation to lesser services, programs, activities, benefits, jobs, or other opportunities;

(6) census data, national polls, and other studies have documented that people with disabilities, as a group, occupy an inferior status in our society, and are severely disadvantaged socially, vocationally, economically, and educationally;

(7) individuals with disabilities are a discrete and insular minority who have been faced with restrictions and limitations, subjected to a history of purposeful unequal treatment, and relegated to a position of political powerlessness in our society, based on characteristics that are beyond the control of such individuals and resulting from stereotypic assumptions not truly indicative of the individual ability of such individuals to participate in, and contribute to, society;

(8) the Nation's proper goals regarding individuals with disabilities are to assure equality of opportunity, full participation, independent living, and economic self-sufficiency for such individuals; and

(9) the continuing existence of unfair and unnecessary discrimination and prejudice denies people with disabilities the opportunity to compete on an equal basis and to pursue those opportunities for which our free society is justifiably famous, and costs the United States billions of dollars in unnecessary expenses resulting from dependency and nonproductivity.

(b) Purpose.—It is the purpose of this Act—

(1) to provide a clear and comprehensive national mandate for the elimination of discrimination against individuals with disabilities;

(2) to provide clear, strong, consistent, enforceable standards addressing discrimination against individuals with disabilities;

(3) to ensure that the Federal Government plays a central role in enforcing the standards established in this Act on behalf of individuals with disabilities; and

(4) to invoke the sweep of congressional authority, including the power to enforce the fourteenth amendment and to regulate commerce, in order to address the major areas of discrimination faced day-to-day by people with disabilities.

Chapter Notes

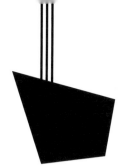

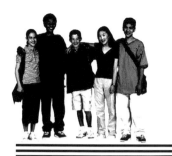

CHAPTER 1

1. Leanne Chilton, *Seizure Free: From Epilepsy to Brain Surgery, I Survived, and You Can, Too!* 2d ed. (Dallas, Tex.: English Press, 2000), 27.

2. American College of Physicians, *Home Medical Guide to Epilepsy* (London: Dorling Kindersley, 2000), 16.

3. National Institute of Neurological Disorders and Stroke, National Institutes of Health, *Seizures and Epilepsy: Hope through Research,* booklet (2001), 10.

4. Quoted in Dr. Donald Weaver, *Epilepsy and Seizures: Everything You Need to Know* (Buffalo, N.Y.: Firefly Books, 2001), 28.

5. See <http://www.academicpress.com/inscight/09231999/brain.htm>.

CHAPTER 2

1. Epilepsy Museum Kork, "The Diagnosis of Epilepsy in the Ancient World," <http://www.epilepsiemuseum.de/english/diagnostik.html#text 1> (accessed April 13, 2002).

2. *The Bible: New Living Translation*, Mark 9:14–27. See also *Revised Standard Edition*, Mark 9:14–27.

3. World Health Organization, "Epilepsy: Historical Overview," Fact Sheet, revised February 2001 <http://www.who.int/inf-fs/en/fact168.html> (accessed April 13, 2002).

4. Quoted in Donald Scott, *About Epilepsy*, rev. ed. (New York: International Universities Press, 1973), 4.

5. Danny Glover, Keynote Speech, Epilepsy Foundation Conference, October 25–27, 2001.

CHAPTER 3

1. National Institute of Neurological Disorders and Stroke, National Institutes of Health, *Seizures and Epilepsy: Hope through Research,* booklet (2001), 57.

2. Christine D. Hagenlocher, "Christine's Challenge," July 11, 2000 <http://www.o-c-s.com/epilepsy/people/cristine.htm> (accessed June 6, 2001, but no longer available September 8, 2001).

3. Alyssa Genna, "Alyssa's Epilepsy Diary," ThinkQuest, 2001 <http://library.thinkquest.org/J001619/diary.html> (accessed April 13, 2002). Reprinted with permission.

4. Epilepsy Support for Youngsters, "My Story by Dania," May 15, 1999 <http://members.tripod.com/~Ted_Bergeron/youngsters-essay003.html> (accessed April 13, 2002).

CHAPTER 4

1. Anthony Hopkins and Richard Appleton, *Epilepsy: The Facts*, 2d ed. (Oxford: Oxford University Press, 1996), 48.

2. Dr. Donald Weaver, *Epilepsy and Seizures: Everything You Need to Know* (Buffalo, N.Y.: Firefly Books, 2001), 49.

3. American College of Physicians, *Home Medical Guide to Epilepsy* (London: Dorling Kindersley, 2000), 29, also see 51–52, n2.

4. Ohio State University Medical Center, "Medication for ADD Being Used as Treatment for Epilepsy," press release, April 23, 2001.

5. Weaver, *Epilepsy and Seizures*, 105.

CHAPTER 5

1. Quoted in Bill Snyder, "Unusual Brain Surgery for Seizures Changes Boy's Life," *The Tennessean*, April 25, 2000, electronic version <http://www.tennessean.com/sii/00/04/25/brain25.shtml> (accessed April 13, 2002).

2. Snyder, "Unusual Brain Surgery."

3. ThinkQuest Message Board, Kristen, "Successful Surgery, No Seizures," April 6, 2000 <http://members.thinkquest.org/mboard/mboard_read.cgi?TEAM=J001619&MSG=477&SID=> (accessed April 13, 2002).

4. Scott & White Hospital, "Luke Potts Learns 'Friends and Faith Are Ultimate Medicine,'" <http://www.sw.org/cmn/potts_l.htm> (accessed April 13, 2002).

5. Kristin Austin, correspondence with author Kathlyn Gay, December 3, 2001.

6. Leanne Chilton, *Seizure Free: From Epilepsy to Brain Surgery, I Survived, and You Can, Too!* 2d ed. (Dallas, Tex.: English Press, 2000), 79.

7. Brian Vastag, "Surgery for Temporal Lobe Epilepsy Is Regaining Favor," *Journal of the American Medical Association* (June 13, 2001), Medical News & Perspectives, 2843.

8. National Institute of Neurological Disorders and Stroke, National Institutes of Health, *Seizures and Epilepsy: Hope through Research*, booklet (2001), 34.

CHAPTER 6

1. Maurizio Passero, "Out of the Shadows," *Talking about Epilepsy* 4, no. 1 <http://www.epilepsytoronto.org/people/talking/vol4/index.html> (accessed April 13, 2002). Reprinted with permission.

2. Pamela, "Talk to Us: Share Your Experiences with Epilepsy," May 28, 2001 <http://members.thinkquest.org/mboard/mboard_read.cgi?TEAM=J001619&MSG=5996&SID=> (accessed November 17, 2001).

3. Alliance for Epilepsy Research, *In Our Own Words*, "Lori Shively's Words" <http://www.epilepsyresearch.org/ourwords.htm#Lori Shively's Words> (accessed April 13, 2002).

4. Quoted in Steven C. Schachter, *The Brainstorms Companion: Epilepsy in Our View* (New York: Raven Press, 1995), 13.

5. Schachter, *The Brainstorms Companion*, 47.

6. John R. McGarrahan, correspondence with author Kathlyn Gay, September 16, 2001.

7. Richard Lechtenberg, *Epilepsy and the Family: A New Guide* (Cambridge, Mass.: Harvard University Press, 1999), 129–30.

8. Joel Davis, "Seizure Alert Dogs: The New Frontier," *Accent on Living* (Winter 1997), 65.

9. Annie Cummins, "Seizure Alert and Companion Dogs: Adam," July 26, 2000 <http://members.tripod.com/~Ted_Bergeron/seizure-dog-essay013.html> (accessed April 13, 2002).

10. Jorie Green, VetCentric.com, "Can Dogs Be Trained to Detect Epileptic Seizures? Maybe, Experts Say," 2000 <http://www.epilepsy.com.au/epilepsy/epilepsyadult.nsf/Content/FeatureStory2?OpenDocument&style=PrintEasy> (accessed April 13, 2002).

11. University of Florida, College of Veterinary Medicine, "Findings to Date," <http://www.vetmed.ufl.edu/ufmrg/dog/dog3.html> (accessed April 13, 2002).

CHAPTER 7

1. Lisa Carney, correspondence with author Kathlyn Gay, November 20, 2001.

2. Kristin Austin, correspondence with author Kathlyn Gay, December 3, 2001.

3. Quoted in Steven C. Schachter, *The Brainstorms Companion: Epilepsy in Our View* (New York: Raven Press, 1995), 39.

4. See <http://members.tripod.com/~Ted_Bergeron/billofrights.html> (site accessed April 13, 2002). Reprinted with permission.

5. Lisa Carney, correspondence with author Kathlyn Gay, November 20, 2001.

6. Kristin Austin, correspondence with author Kathlyn Gay, December 3, 2001.

7. Epilepsy Foundation eCommunities Forums—Dating and Possible Seizures, October–November 2001 <http://www.epilepsyfoundation.org/Forums/messageview.cfm?catid=5&threadid=2218> (accessed April 13, 2002).

8. National Information Center for Children and Youth with Disabilities, Fact Sheet Number 6 (FS6) (April 2000).

9. Elizabeth Goodspeed, "Dating & Epilepsy," *EpilepsyUSA* (September–October 2000), "Between Us" section, no page numbers. Reprinted with permission.

10. Lisa Carney, correspondence with author Kathlyn Gay, November 20, 2001.

11. Jesse, "Not Being Able to Get Jobs, Because of Being Disabled," May 24, 2001 <http://www.epilepsyfoundation.org/forums/messageview.cfm?catid=5&threadid=1197&highlight_key=y&keyword1=jobs> (accessed April 13, 2002).

12. Tim Nourse, correspondence with author Kathlyn Gay, November 13, 2001.

CHAPTER 8

1. Taylor, "Taylor's Story—Life as a Teenage Boy with Epilepsy," May 8, 1999 <http://members.tripod.com/

~Ted_Bergeron/youngsters-essay001.html> (accessed April 13, 2002).

2. American College of Physicians, *Home Medical Guide to Epilepsy* (London: Dorling Kindersley, 2000), 69.

3. Regina Reid, "McEleny Continues Winning Streak with Winning Stroke," *EpilepsyUSA* (July–August 2000): 6, 16.

4. Epilepsy Foundation, "Safer Recreation" <http://www.efa.org/answerplace/safety/recreation.html> (accessed April 13, 2002).

5. John O'Grady, "A Message from John O'Grady," September 19, 2001 <http://johnscharityride.joesacher.com/fromjohn.php> (accessed April 13, 2002).

6. John O'Grady, correspondence with author Kathlyn Gay, November 22–24, 2001. Also "A Message from John O'Grady," September 19, 2001 <http://johnscharityride.joesacher.com/fromjohn.php> (accessed April 13, 2002).

7. Ben Marlow, correspondence with author Kathlyn Gay, November 27, 2001.

8. Terry Ventura, "Jade's Story," The Jade Foundation home page <http://www.jadefoundation.org/jstory.htm> (accessed April 13, 2002).

CHAPTER 9

1. Epilepsy Foundation, "Hormones and Epilepsy" <http://www.epilepsyfoundation.org/answerplace/women/hormones.html> (accessed April 13, 2002).

2. Department of Neurology, Massachusetts General Hospital Web Forum, October 31, 1999 <http://neuro-www.mgh.harvard.edu/forum_2/EpilepsyF/EpilimB.html> (accessed April 13, 2002).

3. Department of Neurology, Massachusetts General Hospital Web Forum, December 8, 1999 <http://neuro-www.mgh.harvard.edu/forum_2/EpilepsyF/HF.html> (accessed April 13, 2002).

4. Epilepsy Foundation, *Epilepsy: A Report to the Nation* (Landover, Md.: Epilepsy Foundation of America, 1999).

5. Centers for Disease Control and Prevention, Office of Communications, "Neural Tube Defects Down by 19 Percent since Food Fortification," press release, June 19, 2001.

6. Centers for Disease Control and Prevention, National Center on Birth Defects and Developmental Disabilities, "Why

Folic Acid Is So Important, Frequently Asked Questions (FAQs)," September 12, 2001 <http://www.cdc.gov/ncbddd/folicacid/folicfaqs.htm> (accessed April 13, 2002).

7. *American College of Physicians, Home Medical Guide to Epilepsy* (London: Dorling Kindersley, 2000), 62.

8. National Institute of Neurological Disorders and Stroke, National Institutes of Health, *Seizures and Epilepsy: Hope through Research*, booklet (2001), 44.

9. National Institute of Neurological Disorders and Stroke, National Institutes of Health, *Seizures and Epilepsy*, 44.

CHAPTER 10

1. Quoted in James Glanz, "A Dream of Fighting Epilepsy with a Flip of a Brain Switch," *New York Times*, January 30, 2001, Science Desk section. Also see James Glanz, "Mastering the Nonlinear Brain," *Science* (September 19, 1997): 1758–60.

2. Charles Marwick, "Research Advances Target Epilepsy," *Journal of the American Medical Association* (June 28, 2000), Medical News & Perspective <http://jama.ama-assn.org/issues/v283n24/ffull/jmn0628-3.html> (accessed April 13, 2002).

3. "Scientists at Children's Hospital and Brandeis Use Video Games to Unlock Secrets of the Brain's Sense of Direction," Brandeis University news release, June 23, 1999 <http://www.brandeis.edu/news/catalyst/complex-systems/epilepsy.html> (accessed April 13, 2002).

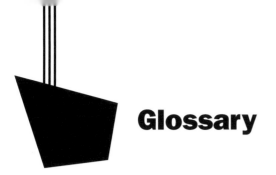

Glossary

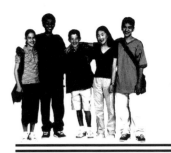

Absence seizure—a generalized seizure characterized by staring or twitching and jerking of muscles.

Antiepileptic drug (AED)—a drug used to treat the chronic condition of epilepsy.

Atonic seizure—a seizure causing a sudden loss of muscle tone.

Aura—a small partial seizure that causes unusual sensations and acts as a warning that a larger seizure is about to occur.

Automatisms—involuntary movements that can accompany generalized or partial seizures, such as chewing, fumbling at a button, or pulling on clothes.

Clonic seizure—an epileptic seizure characterized by jerking.

Complex partial seizure—a seizure that begins in a specific location in the brain that alters consciousness or causes loss of consciousness.

Computerized axial tomography (CAT or CT)—a scan that uses a computer to assemble X-ray images that produce a detailed picture of the brain.

Comprehensive epilepsy center—a medical facility consisting of an epilepsy clinic and epilepsy monitoring unit staffed by neurologists, neurosurgeons, neuroradiologists, neuropsychologists, technologists, a clinical coordinator, and a social worker specially trained to help people with epilepsy.

Convulsion—a seizure characterized by stiffening of the body and jerking, excess salivation (foaming at the mouth), and loss of control of urine, followed by a period of confusion.

Corpus callosotomy—an operation in which a part or all of the corpus callosum is cut, disconnecting the two hemispheres.

Corpus callosum—the network of nerve connections between the two hemispheres of the brain.

Déjà vu—a sense of familiarity, as if an event is repeating itself, which is a common normal experience but may also be part of an aura.

Drop attack—another term for an atonic seizure.

Electrode—a small metal contact attached to a wire designed to record brain waves from the scalp or inside the brain.

Electroencephalogram (EEG)—a test that traces brain waves with electrodes.

Encephalitis—inflammation of the brain.

Epileptologist—a neurologist who specializes in epilepsy treatment.

Febrile seizure—a seizure caused by a high fever in children under the age of five.

Fetus—developing human in the womb.

Fit—an outdated and inaccurate term for a seizure.

Focus—the site in the brain where a seizure begins.

Generalized seizure—a seizure that affects many parts of the brain.

Grand mal seizure—an older term for a tonic-clonic seizure.

Hemispherectomy—a type of epilepsy surgery in which one of the hemispheres of the brain is removed or disconnected.

Intractable seizure—a seizure that cannot be stopped by medication.

Magnetic resonance imaging (MRI)—a scan that uses a large magnet instead of X-rays to form a detailed image of the brain.

Magnetic resonance spectroscopy—a brain scan that measures the brain's metabolism and can detect abnormalities in its biochemical processes.

Magnetoencephalography—a recording technique that measures minute magnetic fields produced by ionic currents in the brain and shows different functions of the brain.

Meningitis—an infection that causes inflammation of the brain lining and the spinal cord.

Multiple subpial transection—brain surgery in which nerve fibers are cut to prevent a seizure from spreading.

Neuron—a nerve cell.

Partial seizure—a seizure that begins in a specific location in the brain, such as the temporal lobe.

Petit mal seizure—an older term for an absence seizure.

Positron emission tomography (PET)—a brain scan that uses an injection of radioactive tracer to measure brain metabolism in order to locate abnormalities.

Simple partial seizure—a seizure that begins in a specific location in the brain and produces an abnormal sensation.

Single photon emission computerized tomography (SPECT)—a brain scan that uses an injection of a radioactive tracer to measure blood flow in the brain.

Spike—an abnormal electrical discharge shown on the electroencephalograph in patients with epilepsy.

Status epilepticus—a condition of recurrent seizures on the same day or prolonged seizures that can be life threatening.

Temporal lobe—a part of the brain important in memory and controlling speech.

Therapeutic drug level—a guide for medication to control seizures.

Tonic seizure—a seizure that causes muscles to stiffen.

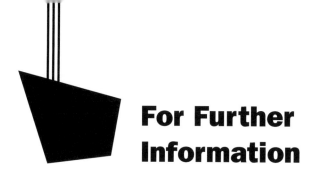

For Further Information

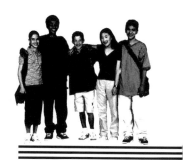

BOOKS

Chilton, Leanne. *Seizure Free: From Epilepsy to Brain Surgery, I Survived, and You Can, Too!* 2d ed. Dallas, Tex.: English Press Publications, 2000.

Freeman, John Mark, M.D., Jennifer B. Freeman, and Millicent T. Kelley, R.D., L.D. *The Ketogenic Diet: A Treatment for Epilepsy.* 3d ed. New York: Demos Medical Publishing, 2001.

Goldmann, David R., M.D., ed. *American College of Physicians Home Medical Guide to Epilepsy.* London: Dorling Kindersley, 2000.

Hopkins, Anthony, and Richard Appleton. *Epilepsy: The Facts.* 2d ed. New York: Oxford University Press, 1996.

Lechtenberg, Richard, M.D. *Epilepsy and the Family.* Cambridge, Mass.: Harvard University Press, 1999.

National Institute of Neurological Disorders and Stroke. *Brain Basics: Know Your Brain.* Bethesda, Md.: Office of Communications, National Institutes of Health, 1992.

——. *Seizures and Epilepsy: Hope through Research.* Bethesda, Md.: Office of Communications National Institutes of Health, 2001.

Richard, Adrienne, and Joel Reiter, M.D. *Epilepsy: A New Approach.* New York: Walker and Company, 1995.

Schachter, Steven C., M.D. *Brainstorms: Epilepsy in Our Words: Personal Accounts of Living with Seizures.* New York: Raven Press, 1995.

——. *The Brainstorms Companion: Epilepsy In Our View.* New York: Raven Press, 1995.

Weaver, Donald F. *Epilepsy and Seizures: Everything You Need to Know.* Buffalo, N.Y.: Firefly Books, 2001.

ORGANIZATIONS

American Academy of Neurology
1080 Montreal Avenue
St. Paul, MN 55116
651.695.1940
www.aan.com

American Epilepsy Society
342 North Main Street
West Hartford, CT 06117-2507
860.586.7505
www.aesnet.org

BRAIN
P.O. Box 13050
Silver Spring, MD 20911
800.352.9424
www.ninds.nih.gov

Citizens United for Research in Epilepsy (CURE)
8110 Woodside Lane
Burr Ridge, IL 60525
630.734.9957
www.CUREepilepsy.org

Epilepsy Foundation
4351 Garden City Drive
Suite 406
Landover, MD 20785

National Association of Epilepsy Centers
5775 Wayzata Boulevard
Minneapolis, MN 55416
612.525.4511
www.naecepilepsy.org

SELECTED WEB SITES

Automated Brain Tutorial
http://home.earthlink.net/~denmartin/brain-map-tutorial.html

Brain Basics
www.ninds.nih.gov/health_and_medical/pubs/
brain_basics_know_your_brain.htm#art

"Epilepsy: An In-Depth Report" (Medscape Health for
Consumers)
www.cbshealthwatch.medscape.com/cx/viewarticle/207626

Epilepsy Circle of Support
www.members.tripod.com/~Ted_Bergeron/

Epilepsy Foundation eCommunities Forum
www.efa.org/Forums/

Epilepsy Menu (a web forum to discuss epilepsy)
http://neuro-www.mgh.harvard.edu/forum/
EpilepsyMenu.html

Epilepsy Resources
www.growingstrong.org/epilepsy/

EpilepsyUSA Online News Magazine
www.epilepsyfoundation.org/epusa/

"Growing Up With Epilepsy"
http://www.thinkquest.org/library/lib/
site_sum_outside.html?tname=J001619&url=J001619/

"Talking About Epilepsy"
www.epilepsytoronto.org/people/talking/index.html

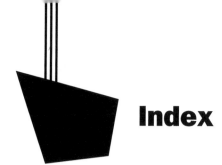

Index

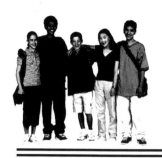

About the Authors

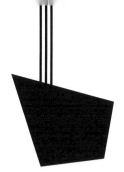

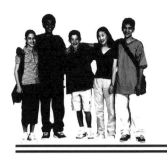

Kathlyn Gay is author of more than 100 published books that focus on social and environmental issues, culture, history, communication, and sports for a variety of audiences. Some of her books have been written in collaboration with family members. A full-time freelance author, Kathlyn has also published hundreds of magazine features and stories, plays, and promotional materials; and she has written and contributed to encyclopedias, teachers' manuals, and textbooks. She and her husband, Arthur Gay, are Florida residents.

Sean McGarrahan was diagnosed with epilepsy at the age of sixteen. He has since controlled his seizures with medication and is now a computer systems integrator working at the Pentagon in Washington, D.C. He applied the information, practical advice, and techniques in this book toward successfully coping with and working through the disorder of epilepsy. A member of The Citadel's class of 1990, he was an award-winning member of the editorial staff of the school newspaper. He currently resides in Arlington, Virginia, where he enjoys bike riding, photography, and paint ball.